Cast Life

NELL JAMES PUBLISHERS
www.nelljames.co.uk

250+ fundraising ideas for your charity, society, school and PTA
by Paige Robinson

Blogging for happiness
A guide to improving positive mental health (and wealth) from your blog
by Ellen Arnison

Birth trauma: A guide for you, your friends and family to coping with post-traumatic stress disorder following birth
by Kim Thomas

How to overcome fear of driving
The road to driving confidence
by Joanne Mallon

Survival guide for new parents
Pregnancy, birth and the first year
by Charlie Wilson

Test tubes and testosterone
A man's journey into infertility and IVF
by Michael Saunders

Toddlers: an instruction manual
A guide to surviving the years one to four (written by parents, for parents)
by Joanne Mallon

The Volunteer Fundraiser's Handbook
by Jimmy James

Cast Life
A Parent's Guide to DDH

Developmental Dysplasia
of the Hip Explained

Natalie Trice

NELL JAMES PUBLISHERS

Published by Nell James Publishers
www.nelljames.co.uk
info@nelljames.co.uk

British Library Cataloguing-in-Publication Data
A catalogue record for this book is available from the British Library.

ISBN 978-1-910923-01-6

First published 2015.

The Publisher has no responsibility for the persistence or accuracy of URLs for external or any third-party internet websites referred to in this book, and does not guarantee that any content on such websites is, or will remain, accurate or appropriate.

Note: The advice and information included in this book is published in good faith. However, the Publisher and author assume no responsibility or liability for any loss, injury or expense incurred as a result of relying on the information stated. Please check with the relevant persons and authorities regarding any legal and medical issues.

Printed in Great Britain.

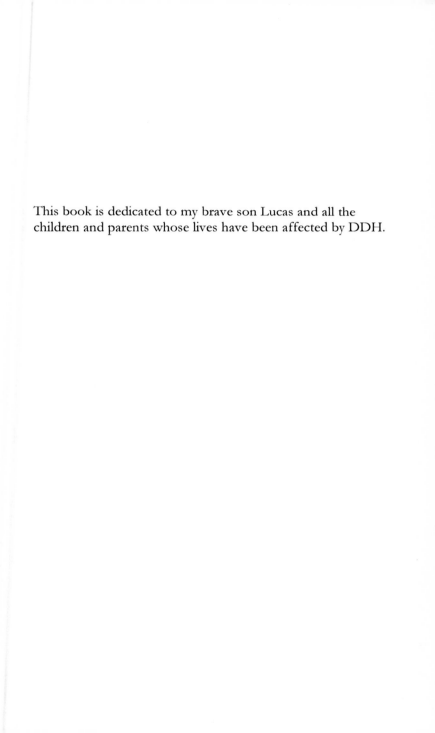

This book is dedicated to my brave son Lucas and all the children and parents whose lives have been affected by DDH.

Contents

Acknowledgements

My brave, beautiful son, Lucas, inspired this book and for that, I thank him. He is my little warrior and I love him deeply. Whilst he didn't have the easiest start in life, he has come so far and I am so proud of his strength and determination. He has more treatment ahead of him but we will be strong for him and together we will get him the healthy hips he deserves.

I would like to send a heartfelt thanks to all of the parents who contributed to this book, for baring their souls, telling their children's stories and offering solace to others. It is the courage and honesty of the real life stories found in these pages that make this book so special.

I thank my husband, Oliver, for his ongoing support and love: I would be lost without him. Not only did he have to watch his son endure operations and months in casts, he cared for our elder son, Eddie, and kept me going without a thought for his own wellbeing.

I am truly thankful that Eddie didn't have DDH. He never once begrudged the extra attention Lucas received and my dear little boy only ever wanted his brother's "dodgy legs" to get better.

I could not have got through the months and years of casts and operations without my amazing family and friends. I will always remember those who were there for me, who held me as I cried, bought me take-away Starbucks when I couldn't leave the house and somehow knew what to say to take the pain away. I know I wasn't the life and soul of the party but thank you for being there for me. I never took it for granted.

Without my cousin, Michele, sharing her lifelong DDH battle with me, I would never have had a true insight into the devastating effects of a late diagnosis. She is braver than many I know, has suffered far too much and is a true inspiration to all.

To have the foreword written by Professor Clarke is an honour and I thank him for his contribution.

I thank all of the experts that offered their time and knowledge to ensure this book gives a balanced and honest view of DDH. With their help I hope I have answered your questions and made things just a little bit easier.

A special thanks goes to Jo Henderson who was my sounding board and proofreader and now knows as much about DDH as me.

Of course you wouldn't be reading the book without the immense help offered by Nell James Publishers, so I would like to say a massive thank you to everyone there.

Thank you for reading this book and I wish you and your family luck and love on your DDH journey.

Natalie

Foreword

Developmental dysplasia of the hip is one of the most common congenital abnormalities. There is a continuing debate about whether there should be comprehensive screening to detect infantile DDH using ultrasound. The diagnosis is commonly made in infancy but often the diagnosis is delayed for many months and sometimes beyond walking age. Whenever the diagnosis is confirmed it is a trying time for parents who are usually unaware of the disorder.

This book explains very simply, but in detail, the implications of the pathology and the need for treatment. This involves splintage but much more interventional procedures in the older child. It is remarkable that there are so few books available to describe this common condition and to assist parents and carers through the very difficult time of splintage or plaster immobilisation and surgery.

This book is a comprehensive guide and will be essential reading for parents and indeed healthcare workers who are involved in the care of children who have developmental dysplasia.

Professor N. M. P. Clarke ChM, DM, FRCS
Consultant Orthopaedic Surgeon

Introduction

Every week, my husband and I stand pitch side in our wellies and watch our boot-clad youngest son get down and dirty playing football.

Whilst some parents gossip and scan emails and others shout encouragement from the sidelines, I intently watch every move my younger son makes with my heart in my mouth and my fingers digging into my husband's palms.

There he is, my little warrior, blond hair, blue eyes and more determination and spirit than many people ten times his age. He runs for the ball as if his life depends upon it and my mind flashes back to the days when those little legs were set rigid in casts and it never ceases to amaze me just how far he has come.

Lucas is my second son and his DDH diagnosis at four and a half months was a massive blow I wasn't expecting. Hearing the doctor utter those words, "Developmental Dysplasia of the Hip", crushed me and filled me with fear for my baby, for my family and for myself. In seconds, our daily lives went from nothing more demanding than coffee mornings and baby massage classes to harness fittings, scans and a constant feeling of uncertainty.

My beautiful little boy has endured more injections and tests, treatments and pain than I care to remember. My nerves have been in tatters and my patience tested, but I was there every step of the way for my child and in a funny way I believe it's made me stronger.

Today Lucas is six, and I'm so proud of him. He loves school, Teenage Mutant Ninja Turtles and his older brother, who looked after him when he had "dodgy legs". After all he has been through, I wish he wanted to play chess or bake cakes, but rugby is his passion and he needs to be the boy he has become and I need to let go of the DDH ghost.

I'm not a medical expert or a qualified professional but I am a mother who has been on the emotionally charged roller coaster ride of DDH and probably have some idea how you are feeling as you read this page.

You might be feeling angry and afraid, wondering what you did wrong and why DDH had to happen to your baby. That's OK. In fact it's more than OK. It's normal and you didn't do anything wrong.

I know the idea of having your baby put under a general anaesthetic is daunting and that having a child in a spica cast is challenging; but I also know you can do it.

When I see my little hero out on the pitch, he is all the evidence I need to believe that whatever shape ball DDH throws at you, you need to grab it by both hands and run for the goal: healthy hips.

I hope you find this book helpful, that it answers the questions you've been wanting to ask someone and that you can take solace in the stories of others and my experience with Lucas, which can be read in full in Chapter Eleven. As well as featuring on my blog (justbecauseilove.co.uk), Lucas also inspired us to create Spica Warrior (spicawarrior.org), a charity dedicated to raising awareness of DDH.

I appreciate there are no images in the book but these can be found on the IHDI, Spica Warrior and STEPS websites. When I started writing this book, I had hoped our story was in the past but unfortunately this isn't the case. We face another hurdle on our DDH journey as our last check-up revealed that Lucas needs more surgery. I hope my words help those still dealing with DDH see that whilst it can be tough, the end destination is worth every bump and blip.

Lucas is evidence that DDH is a journey not a destination.

Natalie and Lucas

Chapter 1: Developmental Dysplasia of the Hip: the facts

Your child being diagnosed with Developmental Dysplasia of the Hip (DDH) can be upsetting, and whilst you may feel a range of emotions, the main thing to remember is that you couldn't have done anything to cause or prevent it.

When Lucas was diagnosed, the first thing I did was head to the Internet. If you can resist, please try not to do this, instead read this book, speak to your medical team and use the STEPS (www.steps-charity.org.uk) and IHDI (hipdysplasia.org) websites. There are also a number of social media forums where those in a similar situation offer help and support.

I don't want to bombard you with medical jargon, but I do want you to be equipped with the knowledge and facts so you can get to grips with DDH and feel as if you have some control again.

What is DDH?
In the simplest of terms, DDH is where the ball and socket of the hip joint fail to develop correctly. It can occur before birth or during the first few months of life.

How does the hip joint work?
The hip joint is a "ball-and-socket" joint. The ball is called the "femoral head" and is at the top of the femur or thighbone. The socket is called the "acetabulum" and this is a part of the pelvis.

In a normal, healthy hip, the head of the femur is a smooth rounded ball, the acetabulum is a smooth cup-like shape and the two sit together like an egg in an egg-cup. Ligaments, muscles and a joint capsule hold them together and promote growth and strength.

In DDH patients the joint doesn't fit snuggly and this means it cannot work or grow correctly.

Typically this condition isn't a one size fits all and if the ball and socket do not fit snugly together there are varying degrees of severity:

- If the ball is not held safely in place, the socket may be shallower than usual; this is called acetabular dysplasia
- Sometimes this makes the joint less stable and the ball may slide in and out of the socket. This is called a dislocatable or subluxatable hip
- If the ball loses contact with the socket and stays outside the joint, it is called a dislocated hip

These are all forms of DDH.

What terms are used to describe it?
Developmental Dysplasia of the Hip (or DDH) is the current medical term for general instability, or looseness, of the hip joint and is the term I have used throughout this book. Other names you may come across in your reading include:

- Acetabular Dysplasia
- Clicky Hips
- Congenital Dislocation of the Hip (CDH)
- Developmental Dislocation of the Hip (DDH)
- Hip Dysplasia
- Hip Dislocation
- Loose Hips

How common is DDH?
According to the International Hip Dysplasia Institute (IHDI), around one in 20 full-term babies have a degree of hip instability and two-three in every 1,000 infants will require medical treatment.

Is there a preferred hip that is affected?
DDH tends to be more prevalent in the left hip and popular opinion is that this is due to the fact that most babies lie against the mother's spine on their left side whilst in the womb. This position potentially puts more pressure on the left hip and causes it to develop abnormally more often than the right.

Does DDH only happen to one hip?
No. DDH can affect both hip joints and this is known as bilateral DDH.

What is the cause of DDH?
In all honesty, there is no definitive answer to this question, which is another reason not to beat yourself up about the diagnosis.

Women release the hormone 'relaxin' into their bloodstream when they are pregnant. This allows their ligaments to relax and also helps the delivery of the baby through the pelvis. These hormones can enter the baby's blood, relaxing their ligaments too and this can make the hip joint loose in the socket.

DDH does not discriminate and any baby can have the condition but the biggest risk factors are:
• A baby born in the breech position
• A baby who was in the breech position in the last three months of pregnancy
• A family history of DDH

Statistically, DDH is more common in:
• First pregnancies
• Baby girls
• Babies with mild foot abnormalities
• If there is a deficiency of amniotic fluid in the womb
• Babies with tortorticollis, a tightness of the muscles on one side of the neck

However, in most cases there is no clear, identified cause or risk and even the most qualified medical professionals cannot predict DDH and do not known why a baby develops the condition.

It is important to remember that whilst predicting DDH is near on impossible, treating it is highly successful.

Is DDH caused by something I did when I was pregnant?

No. There are no precautions that can be taken during pregnancy or delivery that would have prevented hip dysplasia.

How is DDH diagnosed in babies?

Before a baby is discharged from the maternity ward either a paediatrician or midwife will check them as part of the Newborn Infant Physical Examination (NIPE).

With your baby lying on their back, the hips are moved carefully outwards. This won't hurt your child but they may cry in protest. Gentle examinations, known as the Ortolani and Barlow Tests, are used to detect a distinctive click or clunk, which is caused by the head of the femur moving in and out of the socket.

It is important to bear in mind that a clicky hip can be entirely normal and most hips stabilise spontaneously without the need for treatment

However, if a baby's hip is felt to be unstable it will be examined via an ultrasound scan to assess what is happening and if medical intervention is needed. Danielle, a midwife with over 10 years experience, told me:

"Following any type of delivery, a midwife will perform an examination of all babies from head to toe and check their breathing rate, tone and look for serious physical abnormalities. A more in-depth examination of the newborn is then conducted within 72 hours of birth by either a paediatrician or a midwife who has undertaken the 'Examination of the Newborn' course. During this examination the hips are checked thoroughly to look for signs of DDH or 'clicky hip' and appropriate referrals for hip scans are organised if necessary. Indicators such as the baby lying in a breech position or a strong family history of congenital hip problems, lead to a routine ultrasound scan being requested to either rule out, or make a DDH diagnosis.

"In instances where an indication of DDH is made, our job is to offer families guidance, information and support and to ensure that health visitors and GPs are aware of the situation and can do the same."

What is an ultrasound scan and what is it looking for?

Newborn babies' hips are made of soft cartilage which means problems are not always felt when tested by hand. An ultrasound scan is a painless and easy way to get an accurate image of the hip joint. It will pick up any abnormalities as well as show whether the ball is unstable and whether it can move in and out of the socket.

One of the most common and useful measurements of the hips is the 'alpha angle' and this is taken during this simple, painless examination.

For the alpha angle to be considered normal, there needs to be a measurement of more than 60 degrees. Where a measurement of between 43-60 degrees is recorded, mild DDH will be diagnosed. When the alpha angle is measured at 43 degrees or less, the case will be classified as severe DDH.

During the treatment of DDH, the aim is to reach that perfect 60 degrees but do not lose heart if this takes time, it is all part of the journey.

During the ultrasound, the hip is also examined for hip stability and whilst many babies do have loose hips and examiners push at varying levels, in general this shows how far out of the socket the hip will move. The rule of thumb is that 50% of the ball should remain in the socket and where the number is less than 45% there is instability.

Hip instability tends to be far more prevalent in newborns; ligaments tighten as a child gets older. A degree of instability in a six-week old is quite common and sometimes this will be treated and at other times there will be a repeated ultrasound when the baby is around three months old to check what is happening.

Each case is different and your child's case will be assessed and a decision on next steps made by your medical team.

What happens if I have twins or triplets?

In a multiple birth, if any of the babies are in any of the higher risk groups, each child should have an ultrasound examination to check for DDH.

Can DDH be missed at birth?

The answer to this is yes.

The pregnancy hormones that soften and relax your ligaments can stay in your baby's blood stream for a few weeks, making it normal for their hips to be more stretchy and looser shortly after birth and making DDH difficult to detect.

It is also important to remember that DDH may not develop until later in infancy or early childhood. Indications that your baby may have DDH include:

- Deep unequal creases in the thigh or bottom
- Stiff hip joint where one leg does not seem to move outwards as fully as the other – it is often possible to notice this when changing your baby's nappy
- One leg is dragged when crawling
- Legs are of unequal length
- A limp in the leg that is affected
- Abnormal 'waddling' walk if both hips are affected

If you are worried about any of these indictors, make an appointment with your GP who can refer you a Consultant Orthopaedic Surgeon who specialises in treating DDH.

My child is walking and I think there is a problem. What should I look for with regards to DDH?
It is not common for DDH to cause a delay in walking but in some children this is when the condition is first spotted and diagnosed.

Signs to look out for with a child who is walking but you think something isn't quite right include:
- Walking with one foot on tiptoes with the heel up off the floor as a child attempts to accommodate a difference in leg length
- Walking with a limp or waddling gait if both hips are affected is another tale-tale sign of DDH

If you are worried about any of these indicators make an appointment with your GP so that they can refer to a hip specialist for further investigations.

Can I seek a second opinion?
Yes of course you can. Just as with everything in your child's life, you are well within your rights to seek a second opinion when it comes to DDH.

This isn't a legal given but it is your right as a responsible parent.

> "Always trust your gut when it comes to treatment and never be afraid to get a second opinion."
> *Colleen*

> "I didn't get a second opinion because I'm fortunate to live in the same city as one of the best children's hospitals and I trusted our paediatric surgeon's opinion."
> *Sarah*

> "No. It was obvious because her X-rays showed her hips were two inches above her sockets."
> *Sam*

"This is not something that you want to just accept from one doctor because it could have devastating repercussions if left untreated or not treated correctly."
Tina

In my experience, it is best to be sure you understand exactly what your surgeon is suggesting for your child, why and what the outcome would hopefully be. This is an emotive issue and you will feel protective of your child and possibly anxious about anaesthetics, operations and time spent in hospital and casts but do try to keep a level head. Sometimes it is a good idea to take your partner or family member to appointments so you have a second pair of ears and a sounding board post-consultation.

If you have all the facts and still aren't 100% happy, talk to your GP or Health Visitor and see what suggestions they can make.

If you have any questions or concerns, STEPS, Spica Warrior and the IHDI are all great sources of information and can offer impartial advice and support regarding referral, diagnosis, treatment pathways etc.

I have heard swaddling can be bad for baby's hips. Is this true?

Swaddling is an issue over which there has been much discussion in the world of DDH in recent years.

Swaddling is the practice of wrapping babies, from the neck downwards, in a cloth, thin blanket or specifically designed commercial product. It recreates the womb and helps calm babies, stops startling (Moro Reflex) and promotes set sleeping patterns.

Whilst this practice has been used for centuries by many cultures, it is now believed that incorrect swaddling, where the hips and knees are placed in an extended position, may increase the risk of DDH.

A baby is in the fetal position in the womb and their legs are bent up and across each other. The sudden straightening of the legs in a standing position, created by swaddling, can loosen the joints and damage the soft cartilage of the socket.

If you want to swaddle your baby safely, their legs should be able to bend up and out at the hips as this position allows for natural development of the hip joints. Do not tightly wrap your baby's legs straight down and pressed together.

The IHDI has a video demonstrating how to safely swaddle and its official statement summary says:

> "Swaddling infants with the hips and knees in an extended position increases the risk of hip dysplasia and dislocation. It is the recommendation of the International Hip Dysplasia Institute that infant hips should be positioned in slight flexion and abduction during swaddling. The knees should also be maintained in slight flexion. Additional free movement in the direction of hip flexion and abduction may have some benefit. Avoidance of forced or sustained passive hip extension and adduction in the first few months of life is essential for proper hip development."

We did swaddle both our sons and I will never know if this contributed to Lucas' condition. In the haze of a newborn baby and active toddler I am not sure if we did practice safe swaddling at all times and will always wonder 'what if?'

The following method illustrates safe swaddling and ensures that you are doing the best for your baby's hip health:
- Fold back one corner of the cloth to create a straight edge
- Place your baby on the cloth and ensure the top of the fabric is at shoulder level
- If using a rectangular cloth, the baby's shoulders need to be placed at the top of the long side
- Bring the left arm down and then wrap the cloth over the arm and chest and tuck under the right side of the baby
- Bring the right arm down and wrap the cloth over the baby's arm and chest and then tuck the cloth under the left side of

the baby. The weight of the baby will hold the cloth firmly in place
- Either twist or fold the bottom edge of the cloth and tuck behind the baby, ensuring that both legs are bent up and out
- It is important to leave room for the hips to move

Is it safe to use sleeping bags and other commercial products?

There are many products on the market intended to be used for swaddling and these have a loose pouch so the baby's legs and feet are not constricted and allow for natural hip movement.

If you do use them just ensure the legs are not confined or tightened around the thighs and are left to fall naturally.

Are baby carriers, slings and car seats ok to use?

In today's world of parenting, baby carriers and slings are pretty fashionable and have excellent benefits when it comes to bonding as well as keeping hands free when doing jobs and being out and about.

However, it is vital to ensure if these are used, they are used with healthy hip development in mind.

The optimal position for a baby's hips is to be spread naturally apart from one another, knees bent and thighs supported. Many carriers and slings encourage a baby's legs to be held straight, dangling down, or close together (the opposite of the normal position adopted by a foetus). This can, if used over extended periods of time, adversely affect healthy development of joints and soft tissues and place undue weight-bearing stresses through the hips.

Similarly, car seats that are too tight can restrict the position of a baby's hips and prevent them from allowing their legs to naturally fall apart when seated.

Whether it is baby seats, car seats, carriers or slings, these items should all allow your child's legs to remain in, or at least freely move into, their natural position – bent at the knee, turning out towards the hip, the easiest way to think about this is like a frog on its back.

Try not to use any product which forces or encourages your baby's legs to lie or hang straight, or anything which brings your baby's legs in at the knees.

What does the future hold?

The specific treatment for your child will decided by your baby's surgeon based on their:

- Age at diagnosis
- Overall health
- Any other conditions or medical history
- The extent of the condition
- Expectations for the course of the condition

Your concerns, opinions or preferences will also be listened to and every child's journey is different.

Be assured that the goal of any treatment is to keep the femoral head in the socket of the hip so that the joint can develop healthily and function normally.

The need for early detection

Many medical professionals and parents are passionate about the need for early detection and this is not surprising as it can be key to successful treatment and fewer hip problems later in life.

"We are very grateful DDH was detected so early and fixed. My second daughter has had two scans to double check she is ok and we are lucky she hasn't had it."
Claire

"I look back and think I'm glad they found it at such an early age and I have a very beautiful happy daughter."
Antonia

Whilst DDH certainly isn't a matter of life and death, if left untreated it can cause differences in leg length, the development of a duck-like gait, and a decrease in agility, early arthritis and potentially the need for a hip replacement later in life.

"DDH has affected me all my life and I often wonder what things would have been like if it has been diagnosed earlier. Still today too many cases are missed and I really feel for those families dealing with the fallout."
Michele

"DDH is a disorder that is treatable and curable if caught soon enough after birth. The longer it isn't treated, the greater the chance it will become a lifelong, physically limiting, painful disorder that will impact the individual's quality of life."
Anon

"After such a late diagnosis, you never know for sure what the future holds and whether more operations will be needed."
Felicity

"It's frustrating that I still do not have any answers as to why she is like this, why it was not detected at birth and the unknowing of the future."
Sam

"I am now 21 and health wise, I'm not great. I wish things had been picked up sooner and I might not be like this today."
Holly

"I've fought against DDH all my life and I will continue that fight no matter how hard or painful it is. I'm really

frightened of what the future holds and how this will end."
Michele

"Erin is now two years post spica but does not walk as far as her peers. She has leg aches and struggles with her gross motor skills like riding a bike and running. The late diagnosis means we are still waiting to see what further treatment could be necessary in the future."
Emma

There is no doubt that there needs to be more awareness of DDH and education as well as support for those on this journey.

"Scan ALL babies at the six-week check because an earlier diagnosis means less complicated surgeries. My daughter has long-term mobility issues and has to use a wheelchair because of her late diagnosis!"
Felicity

"I believe all newborns should be screened with ultrasound regardless of risk factors. All babies have the potential to be affected and early detection is vital."
Amy

"After everything I have been though, I want every baby scanned for DDH at birth. For children born into a family with a strong history, they must be examined really carefully with no stone left unturned."
Michele

"Stop making DDH a postcode lottery! DDH diagnosis and treatment should be consistent wherever you live in UK."
Sam

"There has to be more information and funding available. We have had to provide all the equipment our child has needed and have not been given any help at all."
Anon

"I know many hospitals and doctors do things differently but there must be a general outline for things that they all follow so we all get the same care and help. A step-by-step guide with tips would be helpful to find in one place."
Samantha

There is no doubt that it is vital for early DDH detection to be made so that treatment can start as soon as possible and healthy hips can be created with the minimum of intervention.

Too many children are slipping through the net and having to endure pain, misery and long-term effects that could have been prevented if their condition had been picked up earlier.

Chapter 2: Dealing with the DDH diagnosis

Being given the diagnosis that your baby has DDH can be an extremely emotional and stressful experience. I'm not sure if you come to terms with it or simply learn how to cope and move forwards, but you do come out the other side.

Whilst the DDH diagnosis isn't terminal and the condition is treatable, many people assume you simply fix what is broken and move on with life. However, this is far from the truth and when the diagnosis is made lives change forever.

> "People belittling what you're going through and think-ing it isn't hard. Everyone seems to 'know' something about hip dysplasia and you'd get comments such as 'it's easily treated', 'well it's not life threatening'. No, it's not and we feel very lucky that it isn't but they're not the ones watching their child in pain after an operation or from cramp in the cast."
>
> *Anon*

> "When I first found out my son had DDH we were all in shock. The GP that referred me to my specialist said to me 'Of all the things that can go wrong with your child this is one of the good things, it will be very in-convenient, but it can be fixed!' At the time I wanted to shout at her how could this be GOOD, but now at the end of the 14 months spica/brace period I can see what she meant."
>
> *Angela*

"Shock is an understatement of the emotions you go through after diagnosis. I had to take a nine-month sabbatical from my teaching career and family life was disrupted for older siblings."
Emma

The main thing to remember is that everyone reacts and copes in different ways. There is no wrong or right way to behave and you will find a way to move forwards that is right for you.

Dr. Rachel Andrew, a Clinical Psychologist who works with children and their families, explains:

"There's no rulebook about how to deal with the news that your child has DDH. Whether they are a few hours old or at full-time school, you'll feel a range of emotions, possibly similar to that of grief, and will handle it in your own way. There may be a sense of loss, feelings of anger, shock, guilt, questions of 'why us?' as well as fear for your child and their future.

"Don't feel selfish about these feelings, they're normal, natural responses. Many parents have an image of what life will be like when they have a child; the clothes they're going to wear, the buggy they're going to buy and the classes they're going to attend, but a DDH diagnosis can shatter those dreams in seconds. It will take time to adjust and whilst it might not feel like it today, or tomorrow, a life based on new ideals will be created, accepted and enjoyed."

Many parents don't know anything about DDH and being told this is happening to their child and family can be difficult. You not only have to deal with the practical side of the diagnosis but also the emotions it brings with it as well as the opinions of others who may brush it aside as a broken bone that needs fixing.

For me, I felt bereft for a long time as well as angry and cheated. I had Lucas in my mid-30s and was looking forward to spending time with my sons, going to the park, enjoying our new home and making special memories. The cute clothes, bath times and skin-to-skin cuddles were snatched away by DDH and I felt huge sadness and grief.

I had no idea how to look after a baby in a cast, I was worried my other son would feel pushed aside and as for being a caring wife and running a PR business, it all seemed too much.

Slowly I got my head around it, I had counseling and addressed these issues and we got to a point where life with Lucas in a cast became the norm. We never lost sight of our goal – a little boy with healthy hips.

Researching and writing this book has allowed me to connect with many parents who have a child with DDH and there really is no rhyme or reason to how you react to the diagnosis and how you move forwards:

"I was distraught."
Emma

"I felt floored! It also came the same week that we discovered our daughter (our only child) has a very rare genetic disorder. We were numb from that news."
Sam

"My advice would be that although it's a very difficult time when you are on the journey try to remember it's not forever. This horrible illness is temporary (apparently as we're still on our journey but I do have to remind myself of this statement)."
Dana

"Sick. Anxious. Depressed."
Karen

"She is my everything and DDH made her even more."
Patricia

"My initial thoughts on Lauren's condition left me heart broken."
Grant

"When you first hear the diagnosis it is soul destroying but they adapt really easily and will amaze you."
Anon

"Just utter devastation. I can honestly say I don't think I've ever cried over anything as much as I did when we received the diagnosis and throughout our daughter's treatment."
Laura

"I was a nervous wreck because I had never heard of it nor did I know what to expect."
Sarah

"We felt total fear, panic and devastation... (rational brain saying it could be worse) but so protective and each thing was terrifying. Once the spica was on, we managed as well as we could and kept positive but finding out was heart stoppingly awful."
Melissa

"Absolutely devastated. I walked out of the surgery crying my eyes out and didn't have a clue what would happen or how it would be treated."
Laura

"Whilst it can be heartbreaking to think about your baby having to have operations and spend time in a cast and you feel helpless about not being able to soothe their cries, know that you are doing the best for your child in the long run."
Anon

"Devastated, shocked, scared and sad."
Sandra

"Felt destroyed when they put the harness on, they handed her back and said 'here you go, get on with it'."
Kerry

"Like my whole world had come crashing down around me, I was in bits."
Gemma

"It is simply another stone that exists in life, which you might trip over, but from which you can simply get up, brush yourself off, and keep moving. At the end of the day, it's a short-term problem with the long-term solution and for that I am grateful."
Heather

"From the way you dress and change your child, to the way they sleep, everything changes and this is upsetting."
Diana

"I thought I would be in tears the first few days but I had done a lot of research beforehand on the Internet and I think I was mentally prepared. I knew what it looked like, usual treatment times, success rates, etc. I just saw it as a challenge and thought "How do I change a nappy? How do I wash her? How can I breastfeed?" I mastered all these things and more!"
Kirsty

"DDH diagnosis is almost a kind of grief itself as you are missing out on the normal things. I missed his chubby legs and squishy cuddles."
Sharon

"To me it was being dealt a bit of bad luck but finding out so quickly just how amazing, resilient and strong children are even as little babies."
Anon

"We saw DDH as something that can be treated and in the end fixed. Yes it's a bind and difficult to deal with at the time on a practical level, but let's not forget there are children with incurable illnesses who cannot be fixed. It's important to stay level headed."
Sam

"How would we prepare for what we were told on that fateful day? We were to have our little one put into a spica cast. A what?!"
Grant

Small steps

You are only human and it may take time to come to terms with the DDH diagnosis and adjust to a life that is dotted with appointments, surgery and time in harnesses and casts for your child.

"Try not to worry too much, the kids take it all in their stride and they got the rough end of the deal."
Amanda

The key to not letting DDH beat you is keeping positive and having a plan. Having been there and knowing when the days got too much, having a positive mental attitude and a vision for the future helped me turn the corner and made all the difference to everyday life. Dr. Rachel Andrew's advice is as follows:

"There are some aspects of your child's condition you simply cannot control, so let go of these and refocus your energy. As your child's main advocate, read up on

DDH, be knowledgeable, ask questions, manage their care and happiness and of course, love them. Don't try to second guess the future, deal with the here and now and you'll be surprised at how well you cope. You may not have asked to go on this journey, but embrace it and try to find good in each day as a positive outlook really helps.

"Having a solid support system is vital. Whether it's family, friends or parents in the same situation, knowing you have someone you can call upon for advice, a cup of tea or a shoulder to cry on is a massive help. If things get too much speak to your Health Visitor or GP. It is healthier to acknowledge your feelings and deal with them than to punish yourself for 'not coping' and remain unhappy. Life will get better, coping mechanisms will be found and you will all survive DDH."

My biggest advice personally is to see your child first and view their DDH as a part of them but do not let it define them. Be just like any other mum; love them, celebrate their achievements, however small, and enjoy what you do have rather than mourn what you don't.

Knowledge is power
Take time to digest what is happening, research DDH and ask questions. The more you find out, the more in control of the practical side of your journey you will feel and in time your emotions will catch up.

Knowledge is power and I certainly found this to be the case when Lucas was first diagnosed and throughout his treatment.

I am not saying swallow an encyclopedia, but learn about DDH and about what your child is going through or might face moving forwards, be clear about their exact condition, the proposed treatment plan and what could come along in the future.

Your brain can only hold so much information so it is helpful to have a notebook, file or Word document where you can keep things in one place as a point of reference.

I still have a folder that contains all of Lucas' notes, forms, contacts, records and X-rays as well as his Red Book and this is a real reassurance. Each meeting we go to I write notes and file them and if there is anything I don't understand I ask again until I am really clear.

From hip angles and operation timings to casts and pain management, there is a lot to learn about when it comes to DDH but you will be amazed at how fast you become a guru about all things hip related.

Family and friends
When you are ready, and not before, let other people know what is happening.

Call them, send an email, ask your partner to tell them but when you do this be prepared for various reactions and have a simple, concise explanation of DDH ready.

Grandparents and other close relatives and even carers may feel the diagnosis acutely and ironically need your support.

There are some people who will find it easy to offer words of comfort, others will try to say the right things but it might not always come out the right way.

Comments like "look on the bright side", "things could be worse" or "at least it isn't cancer" are well meant but they can feel cold and hurtful when you are feeling vulnerable and struggling with what is ahead of you.

There is nothing you can do to prevent this happening, so take your time, try not to hold a grudge, don't be too focused on those blips and in time it will settle and people will find a way to help you as well as deal with their feelings.

"Some family cried all the time, didn't know what to say, others pretended nothing was wrong!! Some friends

stayed away (didn't contact us). You certainly realise who will be there for you all and support you."
Felicity

"Everyone was very supportive but I don't think any of us had any idea how truly challenging this process would be physically and emotionally."
Sam

"Friends and family are supportive although I don't think they realise how hard it can be, the stress of preparing for operations and even appointments really takes its toll."
Leanne

"People cried a lot which made it worse for us."
Fiona

"Our family was concerned and happy to hear about treatment."
Alicia

"Some felt sorry for us. Most people were very supportive. Some brushed it aside saying 'it's just clicky hips'."
Vicky

"Most family and friends were very cautious about what to say."
Krista

"We're very solid as a family, we've been through some very hard times and are good at supporting each other."
Sandra

"We live away from our families so everybody was very keen to keep in touch with us to provide us with moral

support if nothing else - having somebody other than my husband to sound off at or cry to was invaluable!"
Anon

"I met a woman who is now one of my best friends through DDH as her daughter (also special needs) was treated at the same time in the same hospital."
Sam

In time things will settle down, a new pace of life will be found and whatever treatments your child faces, you will have the information, strength and support to get through it.

Let people help

When Lucas was being treated for DDH and was in his casts, I was very careful about who helped me. In hindsight, maybe I could have let more people be involved but I felt like he was my son and it was my job to take care of him.

He was my responsibility and if anything went wrong I would only have myself to blame. So I would struggle to do it all. I now recognise that this was my way of coping and getting through it.

I am not saying go for a wild weekend in Paris but maybe find one or two people who you trust, show them how to safely pick your child up in their cast (to assure your child and them), how to change a nappy and what they can and can't do and then arrange to have some time out.

Having a shower alone and painting your nails, going out for a run or enjoying a coffee in Starbucks can give you the headspace you need.

Online support

Whilst you can find horror stories and nasty photos online, there are online support groups that provide a great way of reducing that feeling of isolation and connecting with other people who are in the same situation.

"Through some Google research I was able to find a few Facebook support groups which provided so much helpful support and advice."
Sarah

"It was such a relief to find support groups on Facebook because even though my family is supportive and I know how much they love my daughter, they just couldn't understand what it was like."
Amy

"Family and friends were beyond supportive and a local Facebook group of mums was fantastic."
Michelle

"The STEPS forum was a great place for my wife to find out if our experiences were 'normal' and led us to meet with other local families which was really helpful."
Oliver

"Facebook groups are where I've made my best friends over the years!"
Felicity

"If it wasn't for two Facebook pages I was signposted to by a local mum, I wouldn't have had a clue. They have got me through this."
Mel

"It was very hard to find a lot of information and I didn't know any families who had been through this so Facebook groups were amazing."
Amy

At the time of writing this book, the majority of online support can be found via Facebook groups but I image that in time other online forums and social media will really help people get support and reach out to one another.

There is no doubt that the Internet is a great place to do research but don't take one site or forum as the only source of information available. Whilst it is great to be able to connect with others, keep stock of where you are and try not to let DDH take over your entire life and friendships.

Outside help

You're not a bad parent for asking for support and given the impact DDH can have, sometimes it is the best thing to do. Whilst counseling and therapy aren't for everyone, it can help you deal with the emotional experiences you are going through.

There's no shame in admitting you need help and sometimes talking to someone outside of the situation can be brilliant. Whether it is the injustice you feel, the anger or simply a feeling of helplessness, do not feel ashamed to ask for help and remember, the stronger you are (physically and mentally) the more available you will be for your child.

Whilst some hospital clinics do have access to psychological or counseling services, your GP or Health Visitor might also be able to help with local experts.

"Being a mum is a hard enough job as it is but to be told your child has hip dysplasia can be tough. As a Health Visitor I help support parents and work with them to find ways of coping and moving forwards. Whether it's a cup of tea and a chat, weekly sessions to look at how they are doing or suggesting they speak to their GP for additional help, be it counseling or antidepressants, the most important thing is that mum feels supported and can cope with a life she wasn't expecting."

Trish, Health Visitor

Medication
If you feel as if you are slipping into depression and simply cannot cope, do go and talk to your GP who will be able to assess if further intervention or medical treatment is needed.

Again, don't punish yourself, speak up and get the help you need to be able to cope with the journey ahead, the more you bottle things up the harder it will be.

Remember: your child has DDH. You don't.

This might seem like a strange comment, but when my husband said that to me in our early DDH days it made me stop and think and put things into perspective.

None of us want DDH in our lives but we have it and as a parent it is your job to navigate the waters for your child and ensure they get the care, support and treatment they need for the end result of healthy hips.

Whilst it might feel like DDH changes things, whatever age your child, your parental role should not be affected. The basic relationship needs to stay the same, and the more positive you can make it, the less difficult the challenge of living with DDH will be.

It is really important that you do not change the way you relate to your child. Whilst you will want to protect them, don't go over the top, remain the same loving, kind, cuddly but firm parent you have always been and this will help keep things as normal as possible. These kinds of changes can unsettle a child, make them think maybe things are really bad and obviously set a precedent for life post treatment.

What to tell your child
Depending on their age you will need to decide what you tell them about what is going on.

When Lucas was diagnosed, he was only four and a half months, what could I tell him that he would understand? The best language at that age (and any age really) is the language of love and cuddles.

As he got older and needed more surgery, it was important for me to use age appropriate language to explain what was happening. Even at age three, when he had his metal work removed, he still had limited understanding of the operation but, of course by then, was scared of hospitals and hated medical staff touching him, so we had to give him a lot of cuddles and reassurance (maybe a bribe or two) that it was going to be ok.

The key here is honest communication with your child to help them deal with the situation. For some children this is a condition they grow up with, a part of their life and therefore at each stage of their treatment you have to deal with it as best you can.

If they are at an age when they do understand what is happening, ensure you explain as much as you can, reassure them that whilst they might feel scared about what is happening and the fact they have to go into hospital, everyone is going to be really kind and help make their legs better.

Whilst you do not want to scare them, being truthful will earn you their trust. If something is going to hurt, don't tell them it won't or they will never believe you again. If something is going be painful, tell them the truth that there might be some pain, or tugging or a sting but that it won't take long, you will be there and they can squeeze your hand as tightly as they like.

Your doctor or GP may be able to give you advice about how best to talk about DDH with your child if you are unsure. Our charity, Spica Warrior, also deals with this.

Walls have ears
One thing to be mindful of is what you talk about when your child is around. Do your best to talk about their condition and your concerns when they are not there, keep any heated discussions away from their little ears. If you need to discuss any issues about their treatment with medical staff either keep it positive and civil whilst they are with you or move to another room.

It is really important that these children feel everyone is on their side, and whilst keeping it together all the time is pretty much impossible; try to remain strong and positive in front of them.

Take one step at a time, one day at a time; I know you can do this.

Chapter 3: Pavlik harness treatment and care

If DDH is caught early enough your child will most probably be placed in a Pavlik harness to see if the hip will reduce, i.e. the ball goes back into the socket.

The Pavlik Harness (also referred to as a splint) is soft and lightweight and offers a non-invasive treatment for babies who start treatment before the age of three months. It keeps the hips in a position to allow normal growth of the hip joint and can be extremely successful:

"My baby was in the harness 24/7 for nine weeks, 23/7 for one week, 22/7 for three weeks, then overnight for two weeks and we're hoping to get the all clear at her next scan. She has responded perfectly to the treatment, we couldn't have wished for any more!"
Kirsty

"My daughter was diagnosed with DDH at birth. She went into the harness at eight weeks old and wore it 24/7 for four weeks. She then went into it for 23/7 for another eight weeks. She has had two follow up X-rays and goes again in a couple weeks for another one. She will be turning one in a few days and has been harness free now for 31 weeks. The doctors say her hips look "perfect" and they were both badly dislocated to start."
Kerri

"My daughter was successfully treated with a Pavlik harness. She was diagnosed at four weeks, in the harness a week later and wore it 24/7 for 14 weeks and at her six month check we were given the all clear. She is now 13

months and has been walking from nine and a half months, which is far better than I ever imagined."
Shirleyanne

A Pavlik harness might seem very medical and constricting at first but once your baby is used to it they really won't know anything else and will settle into it.

For you, the harness can be a challenge in the early days but once you are armed with the facts and have the practical strategies under control, life can go on as normal.

"I didn't see the harness as the enemy but as our friend that would enable my daughter to heal without surgery and spica cast. I was so grateful it had been found so early and that we had this option."
Kirsty

How does the Pavlik harness work?

The harness is made up of fabric straps that fasten around a baby's legs and are held in the correct position by correlating shoulder and chest straps.

Whilst a Pavlik harness is meticulously constructed and meets orthopaedic standards, unlike a cast, it does not rigidly immobilise the hips but instead allows controlled movement by the child as they kick.

The idea is that your baby will be encouraged to rest in a position where the hips are bent (flexed) up to 90 per cent and relaxed out to the side (abduction). In this position the head of the ball (femur) can hopefully deeply mold into the socket (acetabulum), thus stabilising the hip in the correct position for healthy development.

Images can be seen on the Spica Warrior, STEPS and IHDI websites.

What happens to my baby's feet? Will they be left dangling?

The harness comes with specially designed 'booties' that prevent little feet from slipping out of the harness. Socks can be worn beneath the lower leg straps and booties.

My baby only has DDH in one hip. Why do both legs need to be in the harness?

Both legs need to be in the harness as the pelvis is a ring of connected bones; so one hip cannot be correctly positioned on its own.

How long will it take my baby to get used to the harness?

There is no magic number here I am afraid, it differs from baby to baby. Some babies settle straight away, for others it can take between seven to ten days.

Whilst it is hard for us to watch our children struggle and accept that our little bundles of joy look 'different', they are amazingly resilient and adaptable and will never remember any of this. If you do have any concerns or if they simply don't settle, contact your nurse or consultant.

If caught early enough, will a Pavlik harness correct DHH?

There is no guarantee of success using the Pavlik harness but the earlier treatment starts, the better.

How long will my baby have to wear the harness?

There is no set time for a baby to wear this harness. Every single case is different and will depend on your child, their hips and the age at which DDH was diagnosed.

In many cases, babies wear a harness for 24 hours a day for six to twelve weeks with regular checks and follow-up scans.

If these checks show the ball is being held in the right position, there will be a 'weaning' off period when you baby wears the harness for less time each week depending on progress.

If this happens, you will be shown how to take the harness on and off correctly. It is a good idea to take someone with you to see how it is done or even record it on your phone for reference.

During these periods of 'freedom', let your baby enjoy baths, swimming (age and time permitting) as well as movement and harness free cuddles.

It will be up to your consultant to decide a plan of treatment for your baby and it is vital you follow it.

How do I know the harness is properly fitted?
The chest strap should be firm but you should be able to fit four fingers between your baby's chest and the chest band so their chest can expand properly when they are breathing.

The ankle and lower leg straps need to gently secure or hold the legs but they must not be too tight.

How will I bath my baby whilst they are in a harness?
If your doctor has said the harness is to be worn 24 hours a day, then washing your baby in the bath isn't possible, but you still need to keep them clean, hygienic and fresh.

Give them a gentle sponge bath with a soft cloth, paying close attention to their neck, shoulders, groin and behind the knees as this is where their skin comes into contact with the straps. It is also worth paying attention to the hips creases too. Use a clean towel every time and ensure the skin is 100% dry afterwards.

Keep an eye out for any soreness and whilst it is tempting to apply talcum powder or cream, check with your nurse or consultant first, as this can sometimes cause further irritation and clogging.

If your baby is allowed out of their harness for a bath, the steps to follow are:
* Pay particular attention to the skin behind the knees, hip creases as well as the neck and shoulders

- Dry the skin well with a clean towel before re-applying the harness

In both cases, it is a good idea to keep an eye on your baby's skin daily and if you notice any irritation, sores or redness, contact your nurse. The main areas to check are the groin and behind the knees.

Can my baby wear a normal nappy?
Yes, it is perfectly fine for normal nappies to be worn whilst your baby is in a harness. Many people find disposable nappies easier and less fiddly to use than cloth ones and this also means there is less chance of disturbing the set-up of the harness.

The nappy should be worn as normal but needs to be worn under the leg straps for the harness to work properly.

When changing your baby's nappy, never lift them up by their legs as you may have done in the past. Instead support them under their bottom and gently hold their feet together and carefully change them ensuring you keep the hips secure and in place.

This might seem tricky, but once you have done it a few times you will find it becomes second nature and you will probably continue to do it this way even after their treatment. Remember, the nappy is worn underneath the harness so take care not to move the straps whilst changing your child.

What clothes can my baby wear if they have a harness on?
Clothes are one of the concerns that spring to mind when parents think about this condition. With many little outfits waiting to be worn, it can be really upsetting to think that none of them can be used. This is a natural part of your journey so don't worry or feel guilty.

The main thing to remember is that your baby can wear 'normal' clothes and with a few easy alterations, they will be comfortable and happy. If you need to, pop a soft blanket over them when you are out and about to avoid people staring or commenting. This will also keep them warm at the same time.

Sam Bowen, the Founder of www.hip-pose.co.uk, knows everything about clothing a child in a harness.

> "My daughter was just six weeks old when she was diagnosed with DDH. After the initial shock of being told she would have to wear a restrictive harness 24 hours a day for several weeks, it was another blow to be told that she would not be able to wear any of her lovely clothes.
>
> "I have since set up www.hip-pose.co.uk and sell clothes for children in harnesses and casts as well as sharing advice for parents too."

Sam's top tips include:

- A baby in a Pavlik harness is in a 'frog' position and their legs can be flexed and fully extended out to the sides. It is for this reason that 'normal' babygrows and sleepsuits just won't work as those legs are straight down and cannot be extended to the sides
- The only way that ordinary sleepsuits, rompers and babygrows will allow for the harness and leg flex is if they are at least two sizes bigger than what baby would be wearing at that time. The trouble with this is the legs and arms will be far too long and the body will be baggy. In short there is too much fabric
- At Hip-Pose, the sleepsuits and rompers are designed to overcome this issue as the legs are at the right angle to accommodate the leg position and the rest of the garment is the right size to fit baby for his or her age. You may choose 'normal' sleepsuits for everyday around the house wear and something that is designed to fit well for out and about

In that case it really is worth trying the following:

- Buy sleepsuits and rompers two sizes bigger (i.e. if normally in newborn buy three-six month clothes) from supermarkets or cheap retailers. Cut off the feet and any excess fabric from the cuffs and arms of the sleepsuit
- Buy baby vests and bodysuits from supermarkets one size bigger than your baby would wear and cut up from the leg opening along the side seam to about 2.5cm under the arm or where the chest strap sits
- It is also a good idea to use vests with collars if you can find them as they can prevent rubbing on the neck
- In winter, cardigans are better than jumpers as they can be left undone and not restrict the harness straps
- Waistbands of any sort should NOT be worn over the harness as they can restrict the straps and prevent the treatment from working properly. No trousers of any kind should be worn during treatment– even if they look cute. Fashion is not worth risking the consequences!
- Loose legwarmers can be great especially worn under dresses to provide warmth. If buying legwarmers designed for babies, make sure they are not too tight on the leg straps. Adult ankle warmers (often sold by dancewear shops) are good as they are stretchy, loose and short enough to cover baby's legs
- Dresses are the obvious choice for girls as they are loose over the legs. The best designs are empire line or just under the chest and a wide gathered skirt. Front opening or side tie options make dressing much easier
- Choose baby clothes that are made from 100% cotton as they are breathable. Also choose stretch fabrics to allow for leg flex and comfortable movement generally
- Remember outer clothing such as coats, snow suits, even footmuffs should allow your baby enough room to flex their legs when they want to (straight out to the sides!) and not restrict the harness at all

Can I breastfeed my baby whilst they are in their Pavlik harness?

Yes, there is absolutely no reason why you cannot continue to breastfeed your baby whilst they are in a Pavlik harness.

You might need to spend a while finding positions you both find comfortable and where your baby's legs are in the correct position, but otherwise continue breastfeeding as if nothing had changed.

How should I hold my baby? I don't want to hurt them.

Simply support your baby as normal and place your hand between his/her legs to support the cast. Don't be scared. They are still your baby and they need you to be strong and confident when caring for them.

Will my baby be able to sleep in their harness?

This is something many parents are concerned about but again your baby will adapt and they will sleep.

As with current thinking, babies should still sleep on their back and, if you can, do your best not to let them lie on their side, as this isn't the best position for healthy hip development.

To keep your baby warm, especially at night, you can use sleeping bags but go for a size or two bigger in order to maintain the correct leg and hip position and ensure no restrictions or chance of the legs being brought together.

How do I know if my baby is objecting to the harness or there is something else wrong?

There is always the chance that your baby is unsettled because of something other than the harness so it is important to be aware of this. As well as looking for any sore skin also check for colic, a temperature, signs of teething and treat accordingly.

If your baby really won't settle, contact your nurse or consultant.

Can I still touch my baby's legs?

Yes of course you can. Now more than ever they need your love and touch and you must never be scared by the harness or DDH.

Talk to your consultant but you should be able to stretch and play with your baby's legs within the confines of the harness. Not only is this is good exercise, but it can also help with healthy digestion, trapped wind and even your baby's mood.

When your baby is ready, encourage tummy time, as agreed with your consultant. As well as creating an element of normality it also forces the hips out and back.

Can I clean the Pavlik harness?

Babies make a mess and get dirty by nature, so do make sure you use bibs and muslins whilst they are in their harness.

There will be times when your harness needs to be cleaned but if your baby has to be in their harness 24/7, do not take them out due to spillages. Instead spot wash the dirty area with cooled boiled water, then, using a gentle washing powder or liquid, either scrub the affected area with a cloth or small brush. I found a nailbrush really effective. Blot the damp area dry with a towel and it should be clean (or clean enough) once again.

Once your baby is being weaned out of the harness, it is possible to wash it by hand in warm water. If you do use your washing machine, put the harness inside a pillowcase to protect the Velcro and use a very mild powder. Low heat tumble drying can be used but preferably dry in the sunshine and fresh air or put on a towel on top of a warm radiator.

Will my baby be able to move around in the harness, especially as they get older?

When your baby is ready to turn over or crawl, the harness should not hold them back in anyway. You do not need to limit your baby's activities as long as the harness is in the correct position and their thighs stay apart.

How do I know if the harness needs checking?

Most of the time the harness will be absolutely fine and your baby will be happy. Signs that things aren't quite right include:

- Your baby has been growing and their harness is getting too tight
- Red marks appear around the shoulders or chest straps and don't fade or get better
- Your baby has blue or cold feet or swollen toes
- Your baby's feet start sliding in and out of the booties freely

Feel free to contact your nurse or consultant if you are worried about any of the above and they will advise you or make you an appointment.

Are there any side effects connected to the Pavlik harness?

The Pavlik harness is a very safe piece of medical equipment but one thing to be mindful of is Femoral Nerve Palsy. This is a rare condition that sometimes occurs in babies who are in a Pavlik harness.

If your baby has this, they will not be able to kick their leg or move their toes when tickled and it will almost be like their leg has gone to sleep. If you think your child might have this condition seek medical attention as soon as possible.

Will I need to buy a new car seat and pushchair?

Most people find their car seats and pushchairs work fine with the Pavlik harness with legs remaining in the correct 'frog' position when the baby is in them.

One piece of advice is to try and avoid long car journeys on a regular basis, if you can, as the seats tend to hold thighs closer together. If you do need to do this, you may want to consider buying a wider seat, for example the Mamas and Papas Sola or Silver Cross Pop.

A full list of equipment can be seen in Chapter Thirteen.

I like using a sling for my baby. Is this ok?

The general advice, and comment from The International Hip Dysplasia Institute is not to use slings that cause the legs to 'dangle'. A front baby carrier, which supports the whole thigh and keeps the legs apart in a frog position, is preferred.

What happens when my baby grows?

Just like clothes, Pavlik harnesses come in different sizes therefore as your child grows, the harness may be adjusted or changed.

Can I take my baby to be weighed by my Health Visitor?

Yes, this is absolutely fine and it means you are keeping life as normal as you can. The key to this exercise is to know how much the harness weighs so you can take this away from the figure on the scales.

You may also like to find a clinic that is quiet, with a Health Visitor you know and trust, especially if you feel sensitive about other people looking at your baby in their harness.

> "Little things like your Health Visitor doing home checks for weigh-ins whilst your child is in a harness or putting you in touch with other parents who have dealt with DDH can really help."
> Trish, Health Visitor

What happens if the Pavlik harness works?

First of all, celebrate this fantastic news. You may have to have follow-up checks but hopefully this marks the end of your child's DDH journey.

Just as your baby might have been unsettled when they first went into the harness, they may well be the same when it is removed. Life for them will feel that little bit different but it rarely takes long for them to adapt to their newfound freedom. Physically they might remain in the frog-position for a day or so but before long they will be just like any other baby.

Do not be afraid to handle your child normally. This won't hurt them or damage those precious hips you have worked so hard to fix. However, it is advised that you do not put your child in a bouncer or use a baby walker for up to six months after treatment as it is generally agreed that these do not promote the development of healthy hips and may put strain on the joints.

As your baby has spent a significant part of their life in their harness, there is the chance this could prevent them reaching 'normal' milestones but each child is different. Do not worry. They will catch up in their own time and you must not put additional pressure on yourself to keep up with anyone else.

The Pavlik harness didn't work for my baby. What next?
You will have been in constant touch with your consultant and discussing your baby's progress at each appointment so hopefully this news won't come as a complete shock.

Your child will be removed from the harness if you get to the point where your child's hips are not developing as hoped and your consultant will discuss next steps, future treatment options and make the necessary plans.

Whilst this can be tough news, try to keep positive and believe that what you are doing is best for your child.

Key points to remember regarding the Pavlik harness
- A Pavlik harness is used to correct DDH and works by keeping your baby's hip joints in the correct position
- It may take a few days for your baby to adjust to the harness but they will get there and so will you
- The harness should be adjusted as your baby grows
- Clean your baby's skin and keep an eye out for irritation and soreness
- Be aware of Femoral Nerve Palsy
- Be kind to yourself and know you are doing the best for your child

Chapter 4: Surgery

In cases where a Pavlik harness has not worked, or for children diagnosed at six months or older, surgery is generally the next treatment route. However, the thought of surgery can be daunting and worrying for parents and many feel that the lead up to 'the big day' is one of the hardest parts of the DDH journey.

Mr. Hashemi-Nejad, Consultant Orthopaedic Surgeon at the Royal National Orthopaedic Hospital, explains the main surgery options in an easy to understand way that I hope will set your mind at rest and answer your questions:

Closed reduction

The term 'closed reduction' implies that the capsule of the joint (the envelope that holds the hip), is not opened and, although there may be an incision to lengthen the tight muscle, the hip itself is not disturbed.

A closed reduction is undertaken any time after the age of three months up to one year, although some surgeons may consider this up to 18 months. This entails an examination under a general anaesthetic and is usually combined with dye being injected into the hip so that the ball can be seen reducing into the socket. If the ball sits nicely into the socket this may be combined with a small incision in the groin to release the contracted muscles and lengthen them to reduce the risk of blood supply damage to the ball.

The child then goes into a cast. The time spent in the cast varies from six weeks and then use of a hip brace, which continues for nighttime and naptime bracing, depending on how the socket develops. Some surgeons use a cast for three months and occasionally this is in addition to a change of plaster at the six-week mark.

Open reduction

On some occasions, the surgeon may recommend that the hip is too high out of the socket for a closed reduction, or if closed reduction has failed, in which case they may recommend open reduction.

An open reduction can be done through a groin incision, which is known as a medial open reduction. This releases or lengthens some of the tendons on the inner aspect of the thigh, the capsule is then opened and the ball is eased into the socket. The protocol, thereafter, is the same as a closed reduction.

There is no opportunity to do any tightening of the capsule, which is the envelope that holds the hip, or indeed any bony surgery (yes, this is the right term even if it sounds a bit odd) at the time of medial open reduction. Some authorities believe that medial open reduction has a slightly higher risk of blood supply damage (avascular necrosis). Most people do not do a medial open reduction after the age of one, however there are a few surgeons who would consider doing this up to the age of 18 months.

An open reduction through the front of the hip (anterior approach) is the standard way of addressing a dislocated hip. This allows lengthening the contracted muscles. The capsule (the envelope surrounding the hip) is opened, the hip is reduced and any obstruction to the reduction is removed. The capsule is then overlapped, (double breasted), to give more stability to the hip. At this stage, the surgeon may decide whether bony surgery is required to stabilise the hip further. This may involve bony surgery on the thigh bone, known as femoral osteotomy, or bony surgery on the acetabular side (pelvic osteotomy). The child is usually placed in a hip plaster for six to eight weeks.

Femoral osteotomy

A femoral osteotomy is the cutting of the thigh bone below the hip to ensure that the hip is stable in the socket. This can be done at an early age, any time after the age of one year or 18 months, but may also be done at an older age if the hip is not sitting well within the socket and there is a structural abnormality in the thigh bone. The surgeon can cut the bone so they can rotate the bone into the socket or tilt the bone into the socket and the bone is then held with a metal plate and screw. Generally speaking under the age of five, this would be augmented with a plaster because of the child's inability to co-operate with the use of crutches. Over the age of five or six, the surgeon may not use a plaster. The surgeon may also tell you that the plate will be removed at a later date.

Salter osteotomy

In hip dysplasia, the socket of the hip is usually not formed very well. It can grow normally following closed reduction or open reduction if the hip is stable. Occasionally, however, surgery on the pelvis is needed to re-orientate the socket.

The pelvic bone is sometimes referred to as the innominate bone and Dr. Salter, from Toronto, described an osteotomy (cutting of the bone) in 1960. "This is a cut in the bone above the socket and the surgeon can then re-orientate the socket to give improved coverage at the front and the side of the hip to stabilise the ball within the socket."

The surgeon quite often uses some sort of fixation, either dissolvable pins or non-dissolvable metal work. Again, under the age of five or six, Plaster of Paris is used; after the age of five or six the surgeon may choose not to use plaster. The surgeon will recommend removal of metal work at some point in the first year.

Pemberton osteotomy

When the socket is quite large, a Pemberton osteotomy, which is again a type of surgery on the pelvic bone, is undertaken. This allows more redirection and also partial closure of an enlarged socket so that it captures the femoral head. It can be fixed with metal work or occasionally surgeons use bone graft to hold the position of the cup bone. Usually under the age of six, this is combined with a hip Spica.

Chiari osteotomy

A Chiari osteotomy is not usually done at a very young age and it is mainly a later operation. This is undertaken in an older child or an adult where the socket is quite shallow and the hip is irreducible so the socket is not amenable to redirection. If the socket was amenable to redirection the surgeon may suggest a triple or pelvic osteotomy or a periacetabular osteotomy, which are evolutions of the Salter osteotomy with further cuts around the socket to re-orientate the socket.

However, if the hip is not reducible in the socket and the socket is very shallow, an angled cut is made above the socket and the socket is displaced inwardly and the top of the pelvic bone is moved out to give a buttress to the acetabulum. This procedure is very similar to a shelf acetabuloplasty, which some surgeons use to give a buttress to a very shallow socket in order to try and hold the femoral head within the acetabulum.

Every child is different and no two surgery case notes will be the same:

"Pavlik harness worn for 12 weeks. Open reduction surgery at one year and in cast for three months."
Sam

"Pavlik harness, two failed closed reductions, open reduction, open reduction and pelvic osteotomy and brace and still needs further treatment."
Sandra

"First operation (age three) open reduction and pelvic osteotomy and in a cast for 14 weeks. Second operation (age five) open reduction, tendon release and Salter osteotomy followed by a spica cast for 12 weeks."
Felicity

"Open reduction with femoral osteotomy and femoral head manipulated into socket. Plates and pins put in as well."
Gemma

"My daughter had a closed reduction follows by a spica cast for four months. We are in the last month of the spica then she will transition into a brace for a few months."
Sarah

"My child was treated for three months in a Pavlik harness, however this didn't work so they had a closed reduction operation and was then set in spica cast."
Laura

"Our daughter has had two pelvic osteotomies, four femoral osteotomies, pins in her femur above her knee (broken leg), and two hardware removal surgeries. She will need bilateral hip replacements before she is 30 years old."
Alana

"Harness -failed, open and closed reductions both failed, pelvic osteotomy and 10 weeks in hip spica - success."
Collette

"Pavlik harness for 14 weeks. Six weeks 24/7, one week 23/7, one week 22/7, one week 20/7 one week 16/7 then four weeks for night time only."
Kate

"Pavlik harness and Salter osteotomy."
Michelle

"Ultrasound at one day old, which diagnosed DDH. She then wore a Pavlik but it didn't work so at three months she had closed reduction surgery and a hip spica, which she wore for six months."
Claire

"Two open reductions (she had bilateral DD) two femoral osteotomies, two femoral shortenings, and so far one pelvic osteotomy."
Elaine

"Two closed reduction surgeries with plates, pins and spica casts."
Michelle

"Pavlik harness, closed reduction, open reduction plus three months in spica."
Anon

Surgery and complications

Hospital staff will ensure your child is as safe as possible whilst in their care but as with any operation, complications can occur.

A general anaesthetic comes with its own set of risks but this is rare so try not to worry about this too much. Your anaesthetist will discuss exactly what is going to happen, how they will feel, how long it will take for them to go to sleep and any risks before your child's operation.

Other risks that can occur include:
- Patients will often be in pain post-op and relevant pain medication will be given
- Bleeding can occur during or after surgery
- Surgical wounds can occur post-op but do not panic as staff look out for this and are quick to spot any issues. Infections are usually treated successfully with antibiotics but in extreme cases further surgery might be required

- Nerve injury can happen and creates numbness or weakness but this usually heals over time
- Loss of position happens where a surgical correction slips requiring potential additional surgery
- Avascular Necrosis is a condition where a joint is deprived of a good blood supply like the femoral head causing it to collapse but this is very, very rare
- Due to the nature of the DDH procedures scarring can occur. Lucas has a large scar on his left leg but the small incisions from his closed reduction in his groin have gone. Almond and rose oil are both excellent for helping these scars fade once they have totally healed, as is Bio Oil. Do be aware that these need extra sun cream when you are outside as they can be very sensitive

If you have any questions about these issues ask your anaesthetist, surgeon or ward nurses and they will always be happy to help and put your mind at rest.

Surgery and treatment follow-up
Children who are treated for DDH generally need to be kept under long-term outpatient review and your surgeon will ensure you have a plan in place for this.

Chapter 5: Spica casts

I am pretty confident that in your pre-DDH days it is unlikely you would have heard of a hip spica. By the time your child has completed their DHH journey it will be a part of your life, something you appreciate for what it has done for your child and you may even keep it in a memory box when you reach the finish line.

In the simplest of terms, a hip spica is a rigid cast that is used to support, immobilise and protect the hip joint whilst it heals following surgery. The spica covers a child's lower limbs and abdomen and will be set whilst they are still under a general anaesthetic following their hip procedure.

It is worn for between six weeks and three months and in some case will be changed mid-way through treatment but this differs from case to case.

There are four types of spica casts and your surgeon may not know for sure which type your child will have until they have manipulated the joint. You will have to wait until your child is in the recovery room to see just how the cast has been set and what you are playing with.

With all casts, padding is applied next to the skin to minimise the chance of infection and irritation and then fibreglass bandages or Plaster of Paris are wrapped around it. Strips of pink tape are tucked under the edges around the groin area to make it smooth and provide a waterproof covering of the edges of the plaster.

Full Hip Spica

This cast starts from just below the nipple line and goes down both legs to the ankles. Both knees are bent and the child is usually in a semi reclined position.

A bar (often referred to as a 'broomstick') might be built into the cast and placed across the middle to stabilise the legs

Cast Life

and strengthen the plaster. Be careful with this bar and do not use it to lift or turn your child as it may break or damage the cast.

One and a Half Hip Spica
This is similar to the full spica but only one leg is plastered to the ankle (the affected side) and the other to above the knee.

Half Hip Spica
With this model, the plaster starts just under the nipple line and goes down the affected leg to just above the knee. The other leg is left free.

Frog Spica
For this cast, the plaster spreads both legs wide and goes down to both knees and your child really does look like a little frog.

Lucas was in this cast for over three months when he was less than a year old and whilst it was heavy and hid his tiny body, the setting of the cast made it easy for me to lift him and carry him on my hip and protected the work our surgeon had done.

Post-Cast Hip Abduction Brace
When your child's cast is removed, there is the possibility they will be placed in a hip abduction brace for several more weeks. This may also be referred to as a 'cruiser' or 'rhino' brace especially in the US and Australia.

Many children who have been in a spica will lose muscle tone and a brace offers your child's body support as they regain core strength and flexibility. This brace is softer, lighter and far less constrictive than a spica and allows an element of hip movement but it still supports the joint as it heals and grows.

To start with, this brace is placed on your child for 23 hours a day with an hour for bath time and play. Moving forward, it will be used just when they are sleeping. This offers a fantastic sense of freedom and can lead to protests when it has to go back on, but before long, just as with the spica, it will be the norm for them. I would often find Lucas fast asleep on the kitchen floor

66

in his brace, lying on his side with a toe resting on the wall and he seemed very comfortable.

The reality of a spica

Whilst you might be shocked to see your child in their spica cast for the first time in the recovery room and wonder how normality will resume, you will be amazed at how quickly your child will adapt and you all simply get on with it.

> "It was amazing to watch her overcome the blight on her life, walking, jumping, sliding down stairs and being the little girl she always was but in a cast."
> *Grant*

> "Keeping a 12 month old child happy in a spica cast where they can't sit, stand, crawl, or lay on their stomach was challenging."
> *Sarah*

> "At the time, looking after a child in a spica was challenging but I think children cope so well that you all learn to get on with it too."
> *Leanne*

> "I found it challenging to keep the spica clean and smelling fresh. It almost became my mission in life and I would often find myself smelling my child during the day."
> *Anon*

> "The plaster nurse showed us (not very well) how to change nappies. But we don't want to lift her. She's fragile, she may break. Wait a minute she's two and in a cast. How can she possibly be more fragile now than when she was born at a tiny 7lb 2?"
> *Grant*

"The first week in the spica was really hard and it took a little while to figure things out."
Krista

"When she was in spica, we just got on with it. We had to think creatively and keeping a sense of humour helped."
Anon

"Coming home from first round of surgery and new cast with us all infected from hospital with Noro virus! Honestly don't know how we coped but anything seemed easier after that!"
Sam

"Our little one amazed us throughout; she was a star. She walked in a cast, it did not faze her at all. Ever. She was our driving force and inspiration throughout."
Grant

Yes, they might be in some pain following the operation (depending on what they have had done) and feel restricted and uncomfortable in their new 'outfit', but once they have recovered and adjusted, I promise they will astound you.

In the next chapter, I discuss in detail how to look after a child in a spica cast but the key cast care instructions are:

- Keep the cast clean and dry
- Check for cracks or breaks in the cast
- Rough edges can be padded to protect the skin from scratches
- Do not scratch the skin under the cast by inserting objects inside the cast
- Do not allow small toys or objects to be put inside the cast
- Do not put powders or lotion inside the cast
- Cover the cast during feedings to prevent spills from entering the cast

- Elevate the cast above the level of the heart to decrease swelling
- Do not use the 'broomstick' on the cast to lift or carry a child in a spica

Chapter 6: Hospital

When you are discharged from the maternity ward with your baby, the last thing you think you will be doing is returning to the hospital for tests, surgery and cast changes.

Quite often, parents find the lead up to surgery the worst part of the DDH journey because once your child is back at home in their cast and you know what you are dealing with, life takes over and you simply get on with it.

> "Waiting for the surgery date was one of the worst experiences I have ever had to go through. Not knowing what to expect made me imagine all kinds of scenarios. I wondered if my child would react badly to the general anaesthetic; I worried about whether he would hate us; I didn't know what his spica cast would look like."
> *Fiona*

It doesn't matter if it is your first or fifth trip to hospital, it can be daunting for you and your child. As well as being in a medical environment full of new smells and sounds, it can also be very busy and intimidating. However, most stays are only for a short period of time and despite what you feel at the time, they are manageable.

What might seem like a minefield at the beginning, getting to grips with a life that involves hospital visits and stays, soon becomes the norm and after a while you will know the system and almost become a part of the family.

> "I couldn't have asked for a better team of doctors or nurses. She'll have her last appointment when she's 16 and I actually think I may miss seeing them!"
> *Michelle*

Choosing a hospital and surgeon

You can legally choose from any hospital offering suitable treatment that meets NHS standards and costs. It is important to choose a hospital where you feel comfortable and confident and influencing factors for your choice might include:

- How far away the hospital is from your home
- Waiting times
- Parking facilities
- Clinical ratings such as infection and cleanliness
- Availability of support from family and friends
- Personal recommendations
- The reputation of the children's orthopaedic department and ward
- Parent accommodation and provisions such as a kitchen and somewhere to sleep or at least rest

Another important consideration for you is which surgeons work at the hospital you are looking at. Some people go with a hospital choice and others with a particular surgeon and medical team. It is pretty much personal preference and there is no right or wrong here but the following points may help:

- Ask your GP for recommendations and do your research. With this in mind don't be put off by one negative comment. Use your judgment. Also, don't keep searching and searching for a 'perfect' solution as you may go round in circles forever
- Talk to other parents in the same situation and ask for personal recommendations
- Work out the logistics. If you live in Cornwall, a surgeon who is based in Kent might be brilliant but would they be the right choice for you?
- Speak to STEPS and the IHDI as they will be able to offer excellent advice and support

The initial meeting with your surgeon

During your child's first appointment at the hospital you will be seen by your surgeon and your child's treatment plan will be decided from there.

It is really important that your child is under the care of a surgeon you are comfortable with.

> "Our surgeon was lovely. He told me couldn't tell me exactly what to expect - as he has always stressed that every child and every case of DDH is different, but he helped me. It is good to ask exactly what is expected of you, the parent. I was told how to take him into theatre, and how to come and collect him again post-surgery and what I was allowed to do to comfort him immediately afterwards. It helps for someone to tell you what to do in such a high stress situation."
> *Fiona*

> "Our primary support was our orthopaedic surgeon. His nurse then referred us to Facebook support groups."
> *Anon*

> "Our surgeon has been amazing."
> *Melissa*

> "Our surgeon is very upfront and doesn't make any false promises."
> *Gemma*

> "An instant bond was formed with our surgeon. He examined Lauren and then explained her condition. We knew then he would do the operations and that our daughter's condition meant something to him."
> *Grant*

What to ask

Parents can be intimidated by the amount of new information they need to assimilate quickly at the start of the DDH journey. The kind of questions you might want to ask may include:

- Can you explain our child's condition again please and the feedback on the ultrasound or X-rays you have seen?
- What will the treatment involve?
- Can you explain the type and purpose of anaesthesia that is administered during the surgery?
- Can we meet with the anaesthetist before the operation?
- How long will my child be under a general anaesthestic?
- Who will be performing the surgery? You or someone else?
- Do you work with the same team of anaesthetists/nurses/support staff regularly or does it change from surgery to surgery?
- What is the success rate of the operation you are suggesting?
- What kind of cast do you think they will be placed in and for how long?
- Will there be a cast change?
- Will additional casting or bracing be required after the initial post-op casting period? If so, what type and for how long?
- Will there be a bar between their legs?
- How much pain will they be in after the operation?
- What are the risks and possible complications for the procedures you are recommending?
- How long is the typical hospital stay following the procedures you are recommending?
- What are the risks, if any, and how serious could they be?
- Do they really need this operation or treatment?
- What happens if my child doesn't have the treatment?
- How will DDH impact the rest of their life?
- Does the hospital have car seats available and any other equipment for loan?
- Do you know of any local support groups or do you have patients who would be willing to talk with us about their experience with DDH?

- Do you or the hospital have patient education resources about DDH?

If you don't understand something you are told, ask for it to be explained again. Remember this is your child and there's no such thing as a silly question. There is a lot of information to digest but you will be amazed at how quickly you learn and become a walking DDH dictionary.

During your initial meeting also consider the following points to ensure you are happy with the surgeon:

- Do they make you and your child feel comfortable?
- Are they able to answer your questions?
- Do they mind you asking questions?
- Do they put your mind at rest?
- Are they happy for you to contact them outside of appointments and if so how is it best to do that?
- Use your instincts. We have them for a reason so go with them

If you decide to take the private care route, again talk to your GP, do your research and check insurance policies thoroughly.

Relationships with your care team

Once your surgeon and care team are in place, it is vital you build a strong relationship with them. You are all aiming for the same result, healthy hips for your child, so being able to communicate and work together well is key.

> "The NHS nurse treating our daughter for DDH was amazing and became a friend."
> *Sam*

> "I got on very well with my daughter's doctor and I have made friends with the nurses at the hospital too - they are genuinely good people."
> *Patricia*

"Our consultant was amazing."
Kerry

"Care in the hospital was very good and we had an excellent surgeon."
Kris

"We received wonderful support at Southampton Hospital. We are from Jersey so had to fly over each time for cast changes etc. So a lot of hard work but everybody was great."
Ellen

As a parent, you might not be a DDH expert but you are an expert on your own child, and this means you are partners in their treatment plan as well as their physical and mental health.

There is every chance you will feel overloaded with the information being offered to you and it is possible to be intimidated by the medical terms and experts around you, but this is all to help your child, not blindside or trick you.

If you have any questions for your surgeon or nurses, share your concerns and come to an agreement so you feel confident again.

Disagreements
Whilst there will be times when you feel disappointed, frustrated or stressed, try to discuss this away from your child and do not involve them. Don't take it out on the staff – they are trying to help so aim to work together.

If you do have concerns about the course of treatment, medications or even your child's surgeon, work around it calmly, away from your child and agreements can usually be made.

Have your say
A doctor, nurse or therapist must have your consent before they examine or treat your child. As parents, we, of course, want what

is best for our children and therefore it is a good idea to work with your care team and ask questions. This will give you a sense of control.

The law states that you have the right to agree to treatment on behalf of a child up to the age of 18 years for whom you have parental responsibility. However, do note that when children reach 16 years, they can give consent independently.

Explaining things to your child

Depending on what age your child is, it's a good idea to talk to them about why they are going into hospital. This is really important because if they feel secure about the situation, it can make a big difference to their experience.

It is vital to be truthful because this is what will keep their faith and trust in you. Don't say that something won't hurt when it will or they won't believe you again and remember that many children will imagine the worst so try to break that fear down and they will love you for it.

Hospitals can be strange, frightening places for children so explain to your child what being in hospital will be like. Tell them they will be sharing a ward with other children of their own age and that it'll be different from their own bedroom at home. Planning a ward visit can be beneficial for them, and you.

For younger children, playing is a great way to express thoughts and feelings. If your child finds needles frightening, why not play with the blunt plastic syringes you get with medicine or put a cast on their teddy to show them it's OK and won't be so bad, mentioning how fantastic it will be when those hips are healthy!

For older children and teenagers talk things through and make them part of the decision making process. This will give them a sense of control and independence when it might feel as if that is being taken away from them.

Chapter Thirteen has details about some great books that help explain what is going to happen. You could also find family or friends who have been in hospital to talk to them about their experiences.

How long will my child be in hospital?

Children needing surgery for DDH under a general anaesthetic will be admitted to hospital. How long they stay in hospital depends on what treatment they are having, their age and their reaction to treatment.

I am speaking generally, but with many DDH cases, you are looking at a short-term hospital stay of one to three nights.

Plan ahead and be clear about the arrangements and what provisions are made at your hospital. You might be one of the lucky ones who can have a bed in your child's room or on the ward.

In most cases only one parent is allowed to stay overnight, so speak to staff either when you visit the hospital or on the phone to assess what provisions are made for parents and the regulations they have in place.

At our hospital it was one parent per child. I wanted to be with Lucas so my husband stayed as long as he could and either went back home or stayed in a hotel close by in case I needed him. During all of Lucas' inpatient treatments, I stayed overnight. One time we had a private room and I took a blow-up bed. The following time I slept in the chair next to him and on our final visit I was lucky and the next bed was empty – not that I slept much.

Some children's departments now have rooms for parents to stay overnight with their children. Again talk to the staff beforehand and see if this is the case, especially if you are going to be there for longer. You need sleep and hotel bills can add up.

If you have to leave their bedside at any time, ensure the cot or bed sides are up and secure, that they are safe and someone can watch them. I would tend to nip to the bathroom or the shop when my husband was around, but if you don't have this option maybe wait for them to sleep and ask a nurse to keep an eye on them and take your mobile phone with you.

If you have an older child in hospital and are leaving their bedside, let them know how long you will be gone for, and make sure that you are back on time.

Visit the hospital

After our initial assessments and meetings, and before the first operation, we were able to visit the children's ward and meet the nurses at our hospital.

Whilst Lucas was only eight months old, it was reassuring for us to get a feel for what was available on the ward, what facilities were offered on-site and the environment we would be spending time in. On a practical level we were able to test-drive the route from home to the hospital at the time we would be travelling, work out the parking and become familiar with the hospital layout and grounds.

Try to organise this kind of visit before any surgery goes ahead as it can be hugely beneficial and set your mind at rest.

You may also find you need to visit the hospital before the day of the operation for pre-op assessments and tests. Your medical team will inform you if this is the case. This tends to be a pretty quick, routine out-patient appointment for blood tests, swabs, weighing etc.

What to take into hospital

Due to the nature of spica casts, you will need to take the usual items needed for a child's hospital stay, and then some.

I remember when Lucas had his first operation I packed as if we were going on holiday. If only! Whilst I didn't pack the kitchen sink, I did have the steriliser, bottles, dummies and much more as he was only eight months old and I wanted to be fully prepared. However, I wasn't the only one to over pack:

"I took a camping rocking chair. I know this sounds crazy, but we had one at home and I wasn't sure if there would be one at the hospital. My little one was used to me rocking her to sleep so I was nervous to be without

a way to rock her. It stayed in the car because they had a rocking chair, but it felt good knowing it was there if we'd needed it."
Amy

"I made sure I had my child's favourite toy, teddy and blanket."
Carrie

"I took my tablet so I had something to watch whilst Poppy slept (she was in hospital for five days) as I didn't want to use her bed TV in case it woke her up."
Kimberley

"I took bigger clothes, leg warmers, socks and different nappies as I had no idea what to expect from the spica."
Katie

"Snacks! Our hospital cafeteria closed early and we were left with vending machines. Healthy snacks to keep your blood sugar up and help you deal with the stress."
Amy

"I took Rescue Remedy for myself, and healthy snacks for us both."
Fiona

When you are packing, these are the things I would recommend you pack for your child:
- Your child's admission letter and hospital notes. I have a file of everything we have been given since Lucas was diagnosed and take it to each appointment
- Whether they are on your phone or in an address book, have important phone numbers to hand, including your GP's

- Favourite teddy, pillow and blanket. This isn't home but a few creature comforts make a real difference and create a feeling of normality
- Take a variety of books, comics and toys as they will get bored especially pre-op
- Dummies
- Sterliser and / or sterlising tablets
- Bottles, bottle warmer and formula
- Snacks
- Tissues, baby wipes, small bottle of disinfectant, antibacterial wipes and gel
- Photos of family and friends either in a small album or on a mobile phone are great as they can be a comfort for your child and you too
- If your child is still wearing nappies, take a supply in their normal size but also take some in smaller and larger sizes too so you can find the right ones for the spica once it is set
- Room permitting, it is a good idea to try placing sanitary or incontinence pads inside the nappy for extra protection. There are no hard and fast rules here so it is case of experimenting with various makes and sizes to be as water / poo tight as possible

Most people go into hospital with a laptop or a tablet and it can be a lifesaver. As well as having games loaded onto it, your child can watch their favourite TV shows without you worrying about costs or broken TV sets on the ward. It also gives you something to do when they are in surgery and sleeping. Don't forget to take a charger too!

If you find you have too much stuff to keep by your child's bedside, or in their room, keep it in the boot of your car and go back as and when you need it. Better to have too much than not enough.

Packing for you
Remember to pack a bag for yourself and base it on a couple of nights away to be safe.

- As well as a change of clothes and underwear, also pack PJs, an extra blanket, pillow, slippers and socks, toiletries and hand sanitising gel
- Books and magazines are a good idea as well as your phone and charger
- One thing to bear in mind is that hospital wards tend to be kept very warm, so when choosing clothes, lighter layers are a good idea
- You will have your own small locker for your personal belongings. Do not leave any valuables or money by your bed unattended and it is advisable to mark all items of personal property with your name

Food and hospital stays
Jenny Tschiesche BSc Hons, Dip(ION) FdSc BANT, a leading nutrition expert, said:

"The quality and nature of food available for people in hospital varies depending on the hospital and sometimes even the ward you are staying on.

"For this reason and in the context of a child who is recovering from an operation, I would recommend sticking to some simple principles, if you are indeed lucky enough to choose what you are served. Aim for easy to digest protein such as chicken or fish with some cooked vegetables. For dessert, a banana or orange are optimal.

"If you wish to supplement the food available in the hospital, which is recommended due to the discrepancies in quality and quantity as well as the inability to plan meals according to your child's schedule, then here's a useful list of easily available snacks:

- Melon fingers or cubes
- Banana
- Pineapple rings or cubes
- Chicken drumsticks
- Cucumber or carrot batons
- Hummus
- Peanut butter on oatcakes
- Trail mix – seeds/nuts and dried fruit
- Flapjack – ideally with nuts or seeds
- Natural yogurt pots with honey"

The Big Day

"The days leading up to surgery are the worst, no matter how many surgeries your child has had. But every day after surgery things get better. For us it was surprising how quickly things improved."
Sarah

"Our surgeon drew a big black arrow on her left leg, I took a picture that was going to be the last picture I would see of those beautiful tiny legs for a long time. It's a beautiful picture."
Jaz

When you arrive at the hospital for your child's surgery, you will be welcomed by a member of staff and let onto the ward. As well as a bed, your child will be given an identity bracelet to wear at all times whilst they are in the hospital.

Once you are registered, the nurse will explain the processes to you, what to expect, when the surgeon and anaesthetist will be down to see you and in what order your child will be taken down to theatre for their operation.

If your child has been, or is, under the weather, it is a good idea to mention this but staff will ask you this question. Whilst the build up to operation day is massive and you don't want to lose your space on the list, for safety reasons you have to be honest with your medical team.

All kinds of things may run through your mind when it comes to a general anaesthetic and it is only natural to be concerned. The thing to remember is that this is a very safe procedure, but if you are worried then mention it to the anaesthetist who I always found were really easy to talk to and very charming.

Unpack your belongings and try to make your child's space on the ward as much theirs as you can. Try to keep your child's bed area free from clutter so you are less likely to trip whilst you are trying to get to grips with the spica, plus it makes cleaning easier.

If your child has been 'nil by mouth' since the night before, expect them to get hungry, thirsty and grouchy. There are usually toys and games on the ward, with designated areas to play, so try to make the most of these as well as bringing any favourite games, stories and toys from home that might settle them.

Play Specialists are often on the wards and offer activities during your stay. They are full of great ideas for keeping children happy and occupied when they are in their spica too, so be sure to tap into their wealth of experience.

Going to theatre

I personally found going down to theatre with Lucas one of the hardest parts of our DDH journey, and actually one of the most stressful things I have had to do as a parent and I am not alone.

I think that all parents feel some degree of anxiety as they walk to theatre with their child in a gown, often under the effect of pre-meds and knowing when they come back they will probably be in a spica cast.

Don't beat yourself up about this. My husband offered to go with Lucas each time because he knew I found it hard, but as his mummy I felt it was my job and I wanted to be with him. Looking back I am glad I did this but if it is too much and you get too upset, let someone take over. It is a hard time and you are a team.

Most hospitals allow at least one parent to be with their child whilst the anaesthetic is administered. This means you can comfort them whilst they are going to sleep, hold their hand, tell them you love them and kiss them goodbye.

Try to be strong for them. The calmer you are, the more secure they will be.

> "Purdey loved the ride down in the cot, she had all her teddies, a suitcase full of them to be precise, all looking at her from the bottom of her cot. I made sure she had her home comforts and smells around her."
> *Jaz*

During surgery

I found the lead up to surgery the most draining aspect of our hospital stay and after regaining my composure when Lucas went into theatre, I used surgery time to pull myself together and get ready for the next stage of care.

Your child's operation is a good time to freshen up, get something to eat and drink, update family and friends on progress (they will be thinking of you) and, if you can, try to relax. Maybe get some fresh air, read the newspaper, have a look on social media or call a friend for a chat and some moral support.

Leave a mobile number with the theatre team so they will let you know when your child will be in the recovery room.

Words of wisdom from parents who have been in your shoes include:

> "I printed out all of the pictures I had of my daughter and bought a couple of photo albums and whilst she was in surgery I arranged them. It was a great diversion and a great reminder of all the wonderful moments in such a stressful time. It really helped me stay sane and not be a complete basket case while I was waiting to hear how she was."
> *Amy*

"To pass the time whilst our daughter was in surgery, we got something to eat, so we could keep our strength up and went for a wander just to try and keep our minds off things."
Jo

"We went shopping during our daughter's operation to keep us distracted and we bought her a present for when she woke up from surgery."
Kimberley

"To pass the time during the procedure, we got a bite to eat in the cafeteria and had a walk. One tip is to have your mobile with you and make sure you have good reception at all times because our nurses called with updates periodically which helped calm our nerves."
Amy

Recovery

Very often you can join your child in the recovery room when the nurses feel it is appropriate.

Recovery time varies depending on each child, the operation they've had, how quickly they wake up from the anaesthetic, how much pain they are in and medication they need.

I am not going to lie to you here, I don't think you would want me to, but when you see your child post-operation you will feel emotional. On one hand, you are happy they are awake and have come back from the operation safely, but on the other hand, they will be in a spica cast and probably in pain too. Until they are back with you, you won't know what size cast they will be in, how it will be set, how far up their chests or down their legs it will be and whether a broomstick will have been used. Seeing them in it for the first time can be a shock.

You won't be the first and certainly not the last to react by crying but try to keep composed. I know I am asking a lot of you, but remember you need to be strong for them and assure them it is OK.

"As one of the other mothers pointed out to me, you can never be prepared for how it feels to see your child being taken to surgery or seeing them in pain and confused in recovery."
Amy

"I'm not sure anything can prepare you for seeing your baby in recovery, I was a wreck both times she went under anaesthetic but just being there to give lots of cuddles was the best thing for her."
Gemma

"I don't know which was worse - the anaesthetic room or recovery to be honest. I wanted to cry in both but knew I couldn't for her sake (I was heavily pregnant too so hormones were rife making it harder to keep those tears back). Watching your child be put to sleep is terrifying, and seeing them in recovery is so relieving but also heartbreaking as they are so confused and scared."
Kimberly

"I got a fright when I saw my little boy after his first surgery. He was in pain and was absolutely distraught. He was shaking and scared and angry. It was hard to see but my husband and I were together and that helped. I was lucky enough to still be breastfeeding my son at the time, and he breastfed for comfort for almost four hours after surgery."
Fiona

"Coming out of anaesthesia was by far the hardest part for me. She was miserable, inconsolable and nothing I did worked. I wanted to fix it for her so badly, but we just had to wait it out. I tried to focus on if I were miserable, I would probably want my mum to just hold me and be there with me and that, alone, would be comforting even if she couldn't fix it for me. That focus helped ease the process a little bit, just trying to be there for her and not so much fix it."

Amy

Just like adults, children respond to general anaesthestics differently but they are likely to be disorientated, upset, in pain, straining their voices or crying. Having you there to comfort them is really important.

Be as calm and reassuring as you can. The sound of your voice will help settle them as will your touch and smell. When I was in hospital with Lucas, I actually got into bed with him in the recovery room as he was so distressed and it really did help calm him down.

Things to be aware of during the immediate recovery period:

- Your child might have an IV drip when you see them after their operations. Do not be alarmed. This might be to deliver medication or to prevent dehydration but the staff will let you know what it is for and monitor the situation
- Your child may experience pain or muscle spasms and they will be given medication as required. The nurses will keep an eye on the situation in recovery and back on the ward and act accordingly
- As with adults, your child may feel, or be, sick due to the anaesthetic. This should pass, but if it doesn't medication may be administered to ease the symptoms
- Your child may have swelling around the genital area, do not panic. This is normal due to the proximity of some incisions in that area but it should calm down relatively quickly
- You and your child will return to their ward or room once a full assessment has been done. This includes checking of

temperature, pulse, respiratory rate, blood pressure, IV (intravenous line), cast and an assessment for pain

The majority of children recover quickly and whilst they might be tired and foggy for a while, most will be fine. Sipping water will help them rehydrate and once they are fine with that, trying some lunch or tea, depending on when their operation was, is the next step.

When your child goes into a spica cast, there will be a period of readjustment for both them and you. Take your time, ask all the questions you need to and get staff to show you how to care for your child whilst they are in plaster.

If this was a cast change or hardware removal, it is likely you will spend less time in hospital and may be out on the same day.

Remainder of your stay
Once you are back on the ward or in your room, your child will have the following treatment and care:
- Their temperature will be taken regularly
- Their pain and pain relief will be managed as required. This is usually with nothing stronger than paracetamol (ibuprofen depending on the hospital and opinion of staff) however in some cases morphine is used
- The cast will be checked to ensure it fits properly, there is no swelling, no sharp edges and that your child's toes are warm and pink with good blood return

How long your child remains in hospital depends on their age, recovery from the operation and anaesthetic as well as the procedure they have had done. It will also depend on any pain they are in and any infection that might occur.

During the day
Keeping a routine can help your child feel more secure. If you can stick to your usual mealtimes, washing and bedtime routines

with stories and favourite toys and blankets to keep things familiar.

Remember; if you can, to take a break. Even ten minutes for a cup of tea and a breather can help keep you on track. Whether it is your partner, a nurse who can spare five minutes or a family member or friend, ask them to take over so you can duck out and get a little head space.

You will be better able to care for your child and give them the support they need if you are coping well yourself.

"Stays in hospital are hard, tiring and weary. They are however necessary. Don't get hung up on the small stuff. A few nights out your life is well worth it if it saves your son/daughter having a hip replacement in twenty years' time."
Grant

Other patients

It is amazing how DDH families rally together not only on social media and in support groups, but also on hospital wards. You are all busy looking after your own child and everyone is in the same boat, but I have always been staggered how people will simply start up conversations, share stories, get each other a cuppa or look out for your child if you need to pop to the loo or shop. Make the most of this, as it's where lasting friendships and support can be found.

Before you leave hospital

For many of us, we simply want to get out of the hospital and carry on with our lives but it is important to ensure you leave feeling confident that you can cope with the spica and the journey ahead.

Don't worry if you don't think you will cope, you will and so will your child. The staff who supported us were amazing. They were so happy to help and ensure we knew what we were doing and felt confident. The nurses on your ward will show you how to:

- Pick up and carry your child
- Change their position correctly
- Change a nappy
- Use bedpans
- Feed successfully
- Breastfeed
- Bath
- How to use a spica table / beanbag / high chair (if they have them on the ward)
- Give advice on pain relief
- How to transport your child

All of these points are covered further in Chapter Seven.

Wheels

Getting around safely is going to be really key. You will need a car seat that accommodates your child whilst they are in their spica. The two brands that have DDH specific car seats are Britax and Maxi-Cosi. More details can be found in Chapter Thirteen about this.

A buggy / pram fitting may also be carried out by your nurse before you go home and again, you may need to use blankets or towels to get the positioning correct.

Children who are too big for buggies may need a wheelchair to get around and your hospital will help with this.

Chapter Thirteen covers all of this in-depth as well information about grants, loans and suppliers.

What to take home

Take EVERYTHING you took into hospital with you, home again. Sounds silly but in our post-op shock we actually left a bag of clothes and notes at the hospital when Lucas had his first operation and had to go back the next day.

Other items you will want to take home include:
- Any information about spica cast care your nurse has given you

- Prescriptions (filled when possible) that have been given to your child
- Any extra supplies offered including nappies, tape, bedpans
- Any special equipment you are being loaned, i.e. wheelchair, car seat or harness
- Details of the next medicine dosage (amount and time) so you can carry on seamlessly managing pain at home
- The ward telephone number
- Patient notes
- Details of the next appointment
- Phone numbers of other parents for moral support

Surgery cancellations

Be aware that appointments and surgery can be cancelled. This happened to us the night before Lucas was due to have an open reduction and femoral osteotomy. Not only was I disappointed because we were psyched and ready to go on our next leg of the journey, but it also meant I had to reorganise childcare for my other son as well as work plans for us.

I am not saying this will happen to you but just be aware it can happen and you need to be able to go with it as much as you can.

You are not alone at home

Just because you are at home, it doesn't mean you are alone, especially in the early days. If you have any concerns or questions call your ward, plaster room, surgeon or GP.

Facebook forums are great for parents with questions. It is always good to know you aren't the only one going through this and the first few days back at home can generate many concerns.

Chapter 7: Cast life

Whilst no one likes being in hospital, knowing that there's a medical team moments away can be a huge comfort when your child first goes into a spica cast. Once you are discharged and sent home the feeling of new responsibilities, pain and discomfort to manage and a change in your child can be overwhelming.

However, it is amazing how quickly they adapt to cast life and, of course, the calmer and more positive you can be, the happier they will be.

> "Whatever you do, don't make her hate this. Teach her to laugh while stuck in the cast."
> *Julie*

> "I would tell parents new to this journey that a spica cast really isn't as scary as it sounds at first. You would be surprised how quickly babies adjust to the change. Just be patient and do what works for you."
> *Sarah*

> "What I would say is 'whilst their hips are sleeping, exercise their minds, help them laugh, learn and grow'. They are such incredibly resilient beings. I couldn't be prouder of my little boy."
> *Laura*

> "Home after two days and then the learning begins much like a new parent. That's the only way to describe it. But we managed. We learned on the job and after a few days we ventured out shopping."
> *Grant*

"I tell people life in a spica is like having a child with the inquisitive stubborn mind of a toddler and the mobility of a newborn."
Sarah

"Phoebe was amazing, adapted quickly, remained in the most part a happy baby who was totally inspiring. I think we were on auto pilot and tried to make her time in the cast fun and as enjoyable as possible."
Melissa

"Having a baby with DDH showed me how amazing and resilient babies are! Lena still danced, wiggled her toes, and even learned to crawl in the spica cast."
Krista

"Basically the kids get on with it and amaze us. It's the parents who struggle."
Michelle

"Within a few days of the surgery, she was back to her happy self. We were told that it would be harder on us than it would be on her, and they were right."
Krista

"Be prepared in the first week for a roller coaster of emotions but things return back to normal very quickly and your baby will be back to their happy little selves and adapting to the cast. Stay positive. Things improve daily."
Anon

This chapter looks at the practical side of looking after a child in a spica cast and how you can make it fun (really) and get through each day as happily as possible.

Managing pain and discomfort
To be discharged from hospital, your medical team will be confident your child is ready to leave but beware, they might still suffer some discomfort and pain when you get home.

It can be challenging to know what is upsetting your child when they are first in a spica, especially if they aren't speaking. However, just as you did when your child was a newborn, you will soon learn from their reactions and be able to comfort them appropriately. The kind of issues you may come up against initially include:

- Spasms may occur which means their muscles suddenly contract, causing the leg or body to "jump". These spasms can happen for the first 24-72 hours following surgery
- An infection may occur post-surgery, which can be indicated by a temperature
- Your child can be uncomfortable and their position may need to be changed
- They may simply need a cuddle to make them feel safe and secure again
- The cast can be too tight or cutting into the skin. This should not happen as the spica will have been checked before you were discharged from hospital but do check again at home

If you have any concerns, call your child's nursing team on the ward number you were given on discharge.

"We introduced a dummy to help with the pain and found this worked."
Antonia

Wound care
If your child has had an open reduction or osteotomy, there might be a dressing covering the wound in their groin. Once you are back at home make sure you keep an eye on that area, and be extra vigilant for:

- Fluids coming from the wounds (blood or pus)
- A bad smell coming from the wound area that isn't toilet related
- Your child having a temperature
- Redness and a hot feeling around the area of the wound

Spica safety

It goes without saying, and I can't imagine any parent would do this, but a child in a spica cast should never be left home alone or upstairs without safety gates protecting them.

Ensure your child is well supervised, use stair gates to prevent tumbles and 'spica proof' your home as much as you can. When you prop your child up do so securely with pillows, folded blankets, foam and wedges.

Do not allow your child to stick any objects (coat hangers, pencils, coins, erasers) under the cast as this could injure the skin. If your child does put an object down into the cast and you can't remove it, call your surgeon or GP immediately.

Try not to let crumbs get into the cast, as this this will cause unnecessary irritation.

Check your child's toes daily. I did this throughout the day and anytime I was up in the night. They should be warm and pink. When you press on the toenail, it will turn white and when you let go, it should turn pink within three seconds. Your child should be able to move their toes and they should not be swollen.

If anything causes you concern, call your GP or surgeon.

When to call your surgeon

This can be a really scary time and you will have a million questions. Not all of them need medical advice so do talk to your partner, family and friends.

The times to call your surgeon or hospital ward are:
- If your child has a high temperature that cannot be explained by a cold, ear infection or other illness

- If your child has on-going severe pain and medication is not helping
- If there are cracks, breaks or softening of the plaster
- If you notice irritated skin, sores or blisters on the skin around or under the edges of the cast
- If your child's fingers or toes are bluish, reddened, swollen, very hot or very cold
- If your child cannot move their toes
- There is a change in the position of the toes in the cast or the cast looks like it is slipping off
- If there is an unusual odour coming from the plaster, which cannot be explained by poo or wee

Turning and positioning
As you would expect, children in a spica cannot move easily, so you will need to change their position for them and your nurse will go through this with you before you are discharged. A lot of this is going to depend on the age and size of your child as well as the way in which their cast has been set, so this is a guide not rules that are set in stone.

The main thing to remember is that your child's head and upper body should be slightly elevated at all times. Generally speaking you should reposition your child with pillows at least every two to four hours, including during the night, and remember to check their nappy at the same time to ensure you have all bases covered. Positions for children in a spica cast are:

- *Back*: pop pillows under the head, neck and legs and ensure the heels are free of pressure
- *Side*: place a pillow under the head, another behind the back to prevent rolling, and one more between the legs to offer support to the cast
- *Stomach*: place pillows under the tummy and check the toes are not touching the floor by placing a pillow or rolled towel under the ankle of the leg(s) in a cast and supervise at all times

When you change your child's position, check that the plaster is not digging in and is not too tight around the edges by looking at the tummy, ankles, groin and knees.

Ensure your child can move their heels/feet freely after each position change.

Make sure their feet are not pressed into the mattress, floor, beanbag or chair as this could cause pressure sores, especially when positioned on the stomach.

If your child develops a red area on their spine, it can be a sign they need to spend more time on their stomach, check with your doctor if you aren't sure.

Of course older, stronger children will amaze you and be able to get around in their casts so won't be stuck in one place. I was stunned when Lucas started crawling in his broomstick cast and know of other children who have walked, climbed stairs and pushed baby buggies.

The main thing is to ensure you are following the advice of your surgeon, do what they say and if you have any concerns check with them to be sure.

Lifting your child
When your child is in a cast they will be much heavier and more difficult to lift than before they went in it.

> "My son was two at the time when he first had an open reduction and then a spica. I am very small at 5'1" and my son is big for his age. At first, I had a bit of back strain as a result. But it got better quickly."
> *Fiona*

> "Spica care was hard as it was so heavy and bulky and I hurt my back trying to move in an awkward way."
> *Anon*

> "You really don't believe a small child can weigh so much but in a spica cast they can! I have a weak back so

had to make sure I picked him up the right way and that
his cot wasn't too low down."
Oliver

"I have hip problems, so I couldn't change my baby on
the floor. I couldn't carry her in the cast down the stairs
by myself, so we could only go out when my husband
was around."
Kris

The cast will be heavy and it may feel like you're carrying a block
of concrete because they are set stiff and can't move or mold
into you, which you are used to.

Whether you have a young infant or an older child, when
lifting them it is vital to support them and the weight of the plaster. The golden rule is to never lift them under the arms without
supporting the plaster as well because the weight of the cast can
pull on the joints it is supporting.

Aim to keep your child as close as possible to your own
body when picking them up. This helps prevent you hurting or
straining your back and makes your child feel secure. Always use
proper body techniques when lifting your child:
- Hold your child as close to you as possible
- Bend your knees
- Keep your back straight
- Lift by straightening out your legs
- Do not twist at the waist; instead pivot the legs

Older children in a spica can be very heavy so ask your nurse
about equipment such as a hoist and wheelchair. This can offer
real independence, a sense of normality for the child and keeps
you strong and healthy too.

"The Chunc wheelchair was a God send."
Gemma

"We didn't really invest in any equipment, but the car seat and wheelchair were life savers. They allowed us to live as normally as possible under the circumstances."
Laura

Sleep

Many parents worry about how their child will sleep whilst they are in a spica and again this changes from child to child.

When Lucas was in his frog cast at eight months he didn't sleep that well but whether that was the spica, wind or colic, I will never know. I was really worried the second time round as he was an excellent sleeper by then and was delighted that despite it being warm and being in a broomstick cast, he would nap in the day and slept at night. I think he was exhausted from pulling himself around and at times would even fall asleep on the living room floor watching TV.

In the early days it is very likely you will experience disturbed nights due to pain, cramp, itching and the inability for your child to turn over and get comfy. It can be that even the hospital experience may affect your child's sleeping pattern.

Whilst this can be tough as you will be tired and craving sleep, solutions that work for your child will eventually be found and a pattern will develop.

"Sleep in a spica is comparable to life with a newborn. When I am sleep deprived I just focus on making it day-to-day or sometimes hour-to-hour. We know it's only a temporary stage so that's how we make it through."
Sarah

"Set the cot mattress up to the highest level and then add an extra mattress so you don't break your back picking your child up out of the cot (only for little babies who can't roll over yet)."
Kris

"Sleeping was fine as she (and I) just had to accept she couldn't really move in her cot although most mornings as she grew she seemed to manage to turn 180 degrees!"
Claire

"Sleeping was hard at first and but improved when she could roll in her spica which thankfully was after just a few days."
Anon

"When it came to sleeping we used to prop her legs up using pillows so that they were relieved a little."
Antonia

"We've been very lucky as she sleeps really well. Fingers crossed it carries on."
Kerry

"I found it took three weeks for her to be able to sleep in the cast for more than a few hours. Also took three weeks again after the spica was removed for real sleep to return."
Anon

Children in spica casts often fit in their cot or bed but you may need to make some adaptions when you first get home including taking bars off, lowering sides and even placing mattresses on the floor and sleeping close by.

Do remember that your child will weigh a lot more and be mindful of this when you put them to bed and lift them out again. I always thought that a travel cot was ideal because of the soft sides, but trying to lower Lucas into one and keeping a strong back and knees was never going to happen.

Generally knees are plastered in a bent position, so children usually find it more comfortable if a pillow is placed under their knees when they are lying on their back. It is really important to know that when your child's heels do not rest on the bed, pressure sores may be caused, a rolled up towel under the ankle leaving the heel free will help.

> "I slept with my baby for the first couple of nights and this saved having to keep going into a different room."
> *Anon*

> "Sleeping - pop a blanket underneath their feet so that their legs are not dangling in the air."
> *Amanda*

During the night these kids do seem to be able to move. We started the night putting Lucas in a comfortable position and did as much as we could to support his body, yet he was often found balancing one spica clad leg against his cot in the morning.

For older children, or those whose legs are set extremely wide, an inflatable bed or mattress on the floor might be a more sensible idea. Not only is this comfortable but also safe as it takes away the possibility of them falling out of bed.

> "My son has always slept on a mattress on the floor so we just put in an extra mattress next to his original one and put loads of pillows around. The extra mattress was there for me to sleep on in the middle of the night when he needed care. We eventually got him some pressure foam and a foam wedge to ease pressure on his back. He slept on his back while in spica, even though he is usually a tummy sleeper."
> *Fiona*

One other point to remember is that the spica cast can get warm and act like insulation for the body, so your child may need fewer clothes and covers at bedtime.

Nappies and toileting

It is very rare that a hip spica will be changed simply because it smells so, as plaster soaks up moisture like blotting paper, you need to be vigilant and fast acting when there are any spills or leakages.

Whilst the toilet area of a spica is small, the need to keep it clean and dry is huge. Not only does this keep your child comfortable but it also allows the cast to remain dry and do its job.

If wee or poo remain in contact with your child's skin (under a wet or soiled nappy or beneath the edges of the cast), nappy rash and subsequent skin irritation can occur causing distress and pain. The nurses on your ward should give you details about cast care but the steps we used were pretty simple and effective:

- Use disposable nappies rather than natural ones. It is a personal preference, of course, but disposable one are certainly easier to use with a spica cast and generally soak up more mess and moisture
- It is better to use a smaller size nappy to tuck inside the cast and a larger one over the cast to secure it. This is trial and error I'm afraid but it is worth getting it right to keep the cast dry and your child dry too
- Tuck the edges of the nappy inside the cast but make sure they aren't irritating the skin
- A sanitary towel, incontinence pad or cotton wool balls can be placed inside the nappy for extra absorption and to catch any unavoidable accidents
- Frequent, regular checks of the nappy must be made; at least every two hours during the day and ideally every two to three hours during the night
- As well as frequent checks, as soon as you notice a dirty nappy, change it immediately as this will help minimise skin irritation and soiling of the cast
- If your child is ill, has loose bowel motions or if you are having trouble keeping wee from running under the plaster, cotton wadding or sanitary towels can be used to soak liquid

up. Just like nappies, these need to be replaced as soon as they are wet as they can cause skin irritation and moisture in the cast

- Allow the nappy area to be open to air for a few minutes each day. This will decrease the possibility of rashes and skin irritation and even offer your child a little relief and normality

We all do this differently but other top tips from parents in the know include:

"Sanitary pads make fantastic protection for the open edges of the cast and help in the event of blow outs."
Laura

"I used a size smaller than usual nappy and cut off the sticky tabs. When changing her nappy I ensured I cleaned right under the cast with wipes and then dried it all with a towel."
Collette

"The first week of nappies in the spica was really hard. It took a little while to figure out how to control accidents. My hint is to slide a thin piece of flannel down the back of the cast and tape to both ends. It can be removed and replaced whenever there's a blowout, and the cast will still be pretty clean."
Krista

"The cast will smell, don't let this upset you too much. Look forward to that first bath once the cast is removed."
Laura

Bedpans and urinals

If you have an older child, your nurse will show you how to position them on a bedpan so that moisture doesn't come in contact with the plaster. This can be a sensitive issue so take your time and be as empathetic as you can.

To use a bedpan, carefully turn your child on their side and place it under their buttocks. Then elevate head and shoulders with pillows so when they are placed on the bedpan wee doesn't run back inside the plaster. Check between their thighs to be sure the bedpan is properly positioned.

A folded cloth or toilet paper placed on the back of the bedpan will absorb any moisture and spillages, keeping the cast clean and dry. Carefully placing toilet paper in between the legs will also help by absorbing the wee.

Your hospital may provide a stock of bedpans but these can be purchased from chemists or online easily.

There are a number of products on the market that allow a person to wee in a standing, sitting down or lying position without undressing and these are listed in Chapter Thirteen. Again this is a case of trial and error and what works for your child.

> "Don't be afraid to try something other than what the nurses tell you when it comes to routine care. At five my daughter was obviously not in nappies. We were told she'd have to use a bed pan but I very quickly realised that with assistance, she could sit on the toilet."
> *Michelle*

> "With an older child plan ahead, we had a bed downstairs near a loo."
> *Felicity*

Cleaning and washing your child

As a spica cast is not waterproof, baths and showers are out of the question but you still need to keep your child's skin clean, fresh and free of irritation and sores. The easiest way to wash your child when they are in a spica is to go back to basics and top and tail them with a clean, warm, damp flannel or sponge.

Whilst cleaning make sure you check the skin around your child's spine, ankles, waist and shoulders and wherever the plaster touches the skin so you can also check for soreness.

It is up to you how often you do this but I did it after breakfast and before bed as well as after naps. Lucas tended to get sweaty in the cast and I really wanted to keep him as odour free and comfortable as possible. I used gentle, organic products to clean the skin and ensured it was completely washed off before I dried him.

From experience, the first few 'baths' are the hardest mainly because you don't want to get the cast wet or upset your child but it really didn't take long for Lucas to adjust and enjoy this part of the day.

Hair washing

Lucas was in a spica during the summer and his hair would be soaking wet with sweat, so I also had to ensure it was kept clean and tangle free. Ideas for washing hair include:

- Lay your child on towels on the kitchen draining board or units and gently wash their hair over the sink, ensuring you stand in front of their body at all times to keep them safe. I actually remember my mother doing this with my sister 35 years ago when she was in a spica
- There are inflatable hair washing basins that are like mini paddling pools and you can put these on the floor and wash your child's hair as they lie on the floor with towels or blankets as support
- You can let your child lie across a bed and put a bucket on the floor to catch the water as you shampoo their hair

- Washing hair in the garden when it is warm is another idea and good fun. This worked well for us in the hot summer months and Lucas would then lie on his tummy and play with the water with his brother (cast being kept dry of course)

For all of these ideas it is best to have a second pair of hands for the first few goes to gain confidence and to avoid managing spillages and protests alone. Singing songs, getting someone to blow bubbles or playing music whilst you wash hair can make it less stressful and more enjoyable and fun too.

If your child will not tolerate any of these, gently dampen their hair with cotton wool or wipes then pat dry. There are some dry shampoos on the market that you can try depending on the age of your child and the sensitivity of their skin.

Another thing to remember is that as spica kids tend to spend a lot of time on their backs, their hair can get matted and tangled. I found a tangle teaser brush and child friendly, anti-tangle conditioner were really helpful.

Cast cleaning

Keeping a cast clean can be a mission and if your child is on the move in their spica it is never going to be pristine. Life is busy and stressful enough at this time so be realistic and remember that kids are messy and get dirty. Aim to keep the cast as clean as you can (especially around the nappy area) but don't worry about marks and scuffs and don't let it rule your life.

You cannot wash casts but you can use a small brush or damp cloth to deal with spillages. A low heat hairdryer can be used carefully to dry spot cleaning but I didn't ever do this.

You don't want to start spraying the cast with random potions and lotions but a little baking soda mixed with water can help with stains and a drop essential oil can help with bad smells.

"The day we brought her home from the hospital in the cast at six months, she had diarrhea up the back of the

107

cast... I got it clean and now consider myself to be a spica care ninja. I'm thinking of teaching classes in spica care at my local hospital (you know, in all my spare time)."
Kris

"When changing her nappy I ensured I cleaned right under the cast with wipes and then dried it all with a towel to keep it smell free."
Collette

In all the research for this book, this was the funniest story I came across:

"Apparently I had a reputation for having a super clean cast on my daughter, so the hospital staff found it hilarious that it was MY daughter who got a bucket of sand in her cast!"
Kirsty

All of this, and more, is covered in Chapter Thirteen but remember, there are no prizes for clean casts only healthy hips.

Keeping cool

Children in casts do get hot and even more so in the summer months and warm climates.

* Ensure you don't layer up their clothes too much
* Keep them hydrated, but don't over-do it or they will wee all the time
* Use a cool, damp flannel to keep sweat at bay but remember to dry skin near the cast
* An air conditioning unit or fan can be really helpful especially on warm evenings
* Being outside in the fresh air is lovely but remember just because your child is in a spica doesn't mean they don't need

sun cream. Rub in an SPF but ensure it doesn't affect the cast

- Some people do find a 'cast cooler' helpful to manage moisture and heat

Clothing

With a little creativity, imagination and going up a size, or three, you can find easy solutions that work wonders:

"Legwarmers or cut off tights for casts with no bar."
Sam

"Buy clothes a size or two bigger and dresses and onesies are great with the spica."
Brittney

"Older girls leggings for a boy were helpful clothes."
Sharon

"DDH meant I was able to put my 'tomboy' daughter in a dress which was great."
Grant

Sam Bowen, founder of www.hip-pose.co.uk, is an expert when it comes to clothing spica kids:

1. Try to persuade your surgeon to provide a coloured cast (they come in all sorts of colours!) but if not then you can customise it yourself with a layer of cohesive bandage. It is breathable, water resistant and comes in an assortment of colours.

2. Legwarmers are great for both covering a cast and offering a bit of warmth. Your child's legs will be up to twice the width bigger in a cast so some baby or child legwarmers may be too tight to go over them. We sell legwarmers that fit, but adult legwarmers will work as long as they have stretchy cuffs. If your child's cast has a bar or stick between the legs,

then anything going up the leg will stop where it meets the stick.

3. A cheap alternative for legwarmers is cutting down kids' tights and pulling them up the cast, like stockings! You can either leave the foot on or not. Lay the tights down on a table and cut each leg off across the highest point where the top of the leg meets the crotch. This is a quick way of providing a colour change to legs and providing a bit of warmth. Knitted tights will be stretchy enough and are opaque so you can't see the cast through them.

4. It may be possible to fit trousers over a cast if you buy at least two sizes larger than you need (they will be too long but you can turn the ankles up or under). The stretchier the fabric the better, if you can get clothes in a four way stretch fabric then they'll be best. If your child's cast has a broomstick, the only way trousers will fit will be if you are able to open and close the inside leg seam – baby clothes are designed with poppers on inside legs to make nappy changes and dressing easier. The bigger the child, the less likely it is you will find high street clothes with inside leg poppers for that reason. If you can fix this problem, then the trousers are closed with the poppers either side of the stick.

5. Dressing a girl in a cast is definitely easier but even then, the width of the waist in a cast is greater than the size of the child (sometimes the cast stops at the chest) so tops and dresses with an A- Line cut (larger at the bottom than the top) will allow for this, side tie tops & dresses will also allow for some adjustment. You may still want to pull on some cut off tights or legwarmers to complete the outfit!

6. For children in a cast during winter, coats that are bell or A-line shaped will be a better fit over a cast.

Day-to-day living

The prospect of being at home with a child in a cast, as well caring for your family, can be overwhelming for some parents. Remember, children have the ability to live for the moment, which is a blessing when it comes to DDH as they can be in pain one minute and absorbed by a game the next.

It may not always be easy, but if you stick to a routine, keep them occupied and try to ensure they are having fun, their anxiety, stress and frustration can be greatly reduced and life will be easier for everyone.

I personally found having Lucas in the hub of the house, asking friends and relatives to visit us, rotating toys, keeping a sense of humour and full biscuit tin really helpful.

As one parent told me, "anything a child sitting down can do, a hip spica kid can do" and this is so true. Bubble blowing, arts and crafts activities, racing remote control cars and learning something new, all can be done and more.

"Arts and crafts, sticky mosaics, play dates, trips to the library. When it was a hard day we would bring out something new and generally found this helped lift the mood, helping us all to regroup and get in the zone again!"
Felicity

"iPad, painting, lots of visits from friends."
Leanne

"Still to this day people comment on her attention to detail with drawing and her neat handwriting and I believe all that time spent being creative whilst in her cast really helped her."
Sam

"Lots of interactive baby toys and lots and lots of books."
Amy

"Colouring, Play Doh, books, DVDs when at home (anything that can be done sitting at the table). We went

on plenty of trips where she could be pushed around in buggy with plenty to see."
Collette

"I took her to Baby Sensory classes which were amazing as they didn't involve much movement unlike swimming or baby yoga which we couldn't do. We also did music classes together."
Claire

"Encouraged him to do the same as other kids - he was very mobile! Just took more time."
Sharon

"Lots of arts and crafts, movie nights, outside for fresh air, bubbles and reading."
Jo

"Sticker books, games, and although we do want to limit screen time the tablet has been a God send, as was her portable DVD player."
Elaine

"Her favourite activity was for me to cover the cast in a rubbish bag and let her sit and play with a bowl of water since she couldn't take baths, she loved that."
Sarah

"We bought a Duplo train set and the train would loop around her which she thought was brilliant."
Laura

"We were lucky that our OT got us a hip spica table with seat so Lucy could sit up for feeding and art/craft activities etc."
Sam

"Play Doh, jigsaws, preparing for Christmas, reading stories, drawing, going out in the pushchair."
Louise

"My little one spent the summer in her cast and loved being outside. Getting the dog to catch a ball and then bring it back made her laugh time and time again."
Sue

"She now does sixty piece jigsaws at four years old. No problem. The cast made her sit down and concentrate".
Grant

Fi Star-Stone is an author and broadcaster and has some excellent ideas for making life in a cast a little less awful and a lot more fabulous and fun.

Sensory play
Don't let the cast stop play! Pop lots of plastic sheeting on the floor and over the cast to limit the mess and damage and let them get messy. Have fun with coloured cooked spaghetti or one of my favourites – homemade play dough where you add food colouring, glitter, lavender or peppermint oil for relaxing sensory play time! Not only is sensory play a lot of fun, but it also contributes to brain development.

Books
Creating a little reading nook is an ideal way of entertaining your little one and gives them that little bit of independence they need. A simple cardboard box filled with a selection of books is ideal – or you can invest in a non-tip bookcase that's easy to reach when next to your child. Ensure they are comfortable and supported and can easily reach the books, and make the books interesting and bright. Touchy-feely books, pop-up books and lift-the-flap books are ideal, as are books with bright images and words.

Music time

A cast doesn't need to stop the dancing action let me assure you. If your little one loves music, then spending a little on a disco light is ideal for letting them forget about the restriction of the cast and boogie to the beat of their favourite songs. Sit your little one comfortably and supported, dim the lights and pop on the disco light and music. Let them move their arms and head to the sounds. Wave ribbons on sticks, music shakers or even bang homemade drums to the rhythm. An upside down pan and wooden spoon make a great drum, and a plastic bottle filled will dried peas is an ideal music shaker.

The great outdoors

I know mobility is a huge issue and often getting little ones in a cast out of the house can seem like a nightmare, but the benefits far outweigh the challenge. It gets both of you out and about, and if you are super-lucky and have one in your area, there are special needs playgrounds so your little one can still get involved with playing outdoors.

My favourite outdoor activity is a nature hunt looking for wonderful things such as pinecones, feathers and sticks. It doesn't really matter what you find, it's the getting out there that's important. Fresh air promotes well-being and sleep, something your little one may have trouble with while in a cast so anything that aids a restful night is a high five in my book.

A set of wheels

A buggy or pram that works with your child's spica is an essential piece of kit. Not only will it mean you can get out and about but will also help you retain a sense of normality by allowing you to keep up with your usual routine and schedule.

> "Go for walks, the calming affect that being pushed in the wheelchair had on Ava was magical especially when she was struggling to sleep during the day."
> *Laura*

As with so many things with DDH and casts, there is not a 'one size fits all' solution. Long and narrow, super-wide or complete with a broomstick, only once your child is back in the recovery room will you know what you are dealing with cast wise.

What is important is that you find a pushchair that works for you and if it isn't the one you take into hospital, source it when you get home. With Lucas I used an iCandy when he was in the frog plaster padded out with blankets and a pillow to support him. It was heavy but he was comfortable and happy in it. Amazingly, because of the way his second cast was set, he was the perfect fit for our Phil and Teds with just a couple of pillows used to pack out the back.

In Chapter Thirteen, I have listed some of the most popular models people find really work. Maybe go to a retailer like John Lewis or Mothercare and try them out in-store and see what works with your child's cast.

I do stress that once you have found a pushchair that works for your child, it is vital that you ensure they are safely supported and strapped in using the harness.

Be aware of any sticking out legs, watch that people don't walk into the cast and be careful with doorways and walls – they don't move for spicas I am afraid!

I always kept a rain cover in the basket of our pushchair because getting the cast wet is out of the question. If you don't have one with your pushchair, a large rainproof coat, disposable poncho or even a bin bag will do the job – just keep the cast DRY.

Once you have a pushchair that works for your child's cast (see Chapter Thirteen), there is no reason for you not to get out and about as you did before DDH snapped at your heels.

If you are parking the car, and don't have a Blue Badge (see Chapter Thirteen) be mindful of where you park to make your life easier. Trying to get your child in or out of the car will become second nature for you (and your back) but not everyone will realise the precious load you are carrying so think ahead to make life easy and as stress free as possible.

Look for larger parent spaces and end spaces in public car parks. When parking on the road, ensure your child's door opens onto the pavement rather than the road so you can take your time getting them out.

> "When visiting the hospital after a physio appointment, someone had parked their car so close to mine that I couldn't squeeze her into the gap to get her into her car seat! I just stood in the car park in tears until a kind lady came over to see if I was okay and she kept an eye on Daisy in her pram so that I could pull the car forward enough to be able to get her in the seat."
> *Emma*

Strangers and staring
Staring is a common problem for parents whose children are noticeably different and a spica cast is unusual. Remember not everyone who stares at your child is thinking bad things about them or you.

Some are interested, curious or want to help but a small minority may be rude and ignorant and there is no way to stop the looks, it is human nature.

> "People stared, which I found hard to deal with if I was having a bad day but then some people also just asked instead of just staring."
> *Gemma*

> "Strangers just looked and stared, especially in the buggy! I had to have someone with me when we went for walks as I wasn't very good at dealing with strangers staring."
> *Sam*

> "Strangers sometimes commented about us having a blue badge because it didn't look like we needed it; some

made comments about we must have done something to break both her legs."
Felicity

"I hated the stares people gave us - as if we had injured our child and that's why she was in a cast."
Sam

"The looks grated on me. This has changed my outlook on life and I never ever look twice at anything that doesn't fit society's norm."
Grant

"Strangers were sometimes hard to deal with as I encountered questions such as "What did you do to your child?" and "What on earth is that?"
Claire

"I found it hard that people would stare. I actually had a couple of people ask if I had dropped my baby. As a first time mum I was devastated on so many levels."
Laura

"When I took her to the clinic to have her weighed other parents used to stare at us, which I found very distressing."
Emma

"We have experienced some odd looks and overheard someone say 'how awful for a baby to have broken legs' and I had to put them right! People sometimes look at you like you are terrible for letting your child break their legs. I would much rather people asked."
Bridgette

As well as looking, strangers might ask questions too so it can be a good idea you have a quick, one fits all answer you can give confidently and walk on.

> "Strangers did ask about the cast and when I explained they usually knew someone else who has had it."
> *Kirsty*

> "Strangers always stared or asked what happen and I would tell them."
> *Brittney*

> "Some strangers stared but most were just curious. More people than I thought knew someone who had DDH."
> *Gemma*

> "If someone asked what was wrong, I made every effort to educate them. What really cheered me up was people sharing their experiences."
> *Grant*

> "Some strangers know about DDH and will talk to you, which is nice."
> *Bridgette*

Whatever anyone says or does, this isn't your fault and you need to keep strong for yourself and your child. You can try and grow a thicker skin, stare or actually talk to those people who look and explain what is wrong.

If you feel self-conscious or vulnerable just place a pretty blanket over your child's cast as you would anyway and carry on as normal. Do not let it put you off going out.

I know this can be really hard to do when you feel exposed and defensive on behalf of your child but you will be amazed at how many kind people there are out there and how many have a DDH story.

Returning to nursery and school

The age of your child, the condition they have and your personal circumstances will have an influence over whether your child attends nursery or school whilst in their spica cast.

All mainstream schools and most nurseries should have a designated member of staff who is responsible for special educational needs and will work with parents, teachers and professionals to co-ordinate any additional support your child may need whilst in their spica.

The Family and Childcare Trust (listed in Chapter Thirteen) will be able to help with this and assist with any issues and how to challenge unfair decisions.

You will, of course, need to explain your child's care regarding the cast, listing their needs. It is vital the nursery understands what your child can and can't do as well as knowing how to lift and change them safely. Ensure they have details of their hospital and surgeon in case they cannot contact a next of kin in an emergency.

It is a huge leap of faith for you and a big responsibility for them but if you work together it can be done.

"We were in a specialist nursery twice a week (part of the hospital due to her special needs) and they coped with her in cast brilliantly. The mainstream nursery we had chosen before birth refused to accept her in cast."
Samantha

"Nursery took our daughter back in a week after her operation and brought in additional equipment to accommodate. Fantastic."
Anon

"I work in a day nursery so my daughter came to work with me. I showed all the other ladies how to care for my daughter and they were brilliant."
Leanne

"We could not get our daughter into nursery as she was 'a fire hazard' apparently."
Anon

"When she had to start nursery in the spica they were amazing, so helpful and great at caring for her."
Sandra

"We chose the nursery because they had experience of looking after a child in a spica cast. They went out of their way to make sure my daughter was well cared for."
Trish

"Our nursery was ace. They got a spica chair, had training from community nurses and encouraged our daughter to join in."
Anon

"Nursery were awesome, took training after hours from our hospital regarding lifting, carrying, changing nappies etc. Did everything they could to get her back to her friends."
Elaine

"Our childminder and crèche were excellent at being fully involved and making my son comfortable."
Mel

"Amazing. They accessed money through the SENCO, sorted out access for her and her buggy, all staff

watched the STEPS DVD and organised inclusive activities. While she was in hospital they did a project on hospitals with the other kids and hand delivered a box full of handmade cards, biscuits and toys for her. She loved going back to nursery in her cast and later with her walking frame. They were also brilliant with an emotional mother!"
Claire

"The school was very helpful and I met them before she started. Her friends pushed her wheelchair when she used it, the nurse helped her in the bathroom, a teacher met her so she didn't fall on the steps. When she got the cast off, they were all extra careful to ensure that she didn't fall or get hurt."
Michelle

Behaviour changes and relationships
Just as there are a lot of changes going on in your life, the same is happening for your child and they simply won't know how to process it all.

Sound familiar?

There is absolutely no way of knowing how your child will react to going into a cast. They may become more aggressive, angry or withdrawn, tearful and clingy and this is often because they don't have the vocabulary and communication skills to express their feelings any other way.

Dr. Rachel Andrew, a Clinical Psychologist who works with children and their families, said, "There is no doubt that some children will experience trauma during their DDH journey, each will react differently and whilst some will be fine, others may be more demanding and others might develop post-traumatic stress disorder (PTSD). The main thing to remember in each case is to ensure your child's basic needs are being met and they feel as safe and secure as possible.

"It is key to have a calm home environment with a set routine so your child knows what to expect day to day and try not to sway from this too much. Whilst you may need to play around with bedtimes and adjust travel times, find a way of keeping things normal when their legs and bodies are anything but.

"Have realistic expectations for your child's age and work out what is caused by the situation and what is just part of their development and age. Praise good behaviour and set boundaries and consequences when things get out of hand."

Chapter 8: Diet and cast life

Food and eating is another area that causes parents anxiety and worry, but for many people things don't change at all.

Ideally you should feed your child in as upright position as possible, this may take a few tries to get right depending on the cast setting. Whether you use a highchair, spica table, buggy, wheelchair or someone's lap, ensure they are safe, secure and happy.

> "Having a spica chair allowed my daughter to sit and feed herself, if she hadn't been able to do this, I don't think she would have eaten."
> *Sam*

> "She happily sat in her Chico Happy Snack chair for meals."
> *Anon*

Rather than offering three square meals a day, try smaller, more frequent ones because the plaster can be tight around the tummy and make children feel full quickly.

> "My little one loves eating cubes of cheese, raisins and lots of finger foods that don't make too many crumbs."
> *Maddy*

> "Small, frequent meals of easy to digest food worked for us and lots of drinks, especially water."
> *Sam*

Keep the food healthy, don't use sugary snacks as rewards, be calm and the rest will follow.

"My daughter continued to eat what the rest of the family did at mealtime plus her usual snacks"
Susan

"Her favourite things were strawberries and pasta and nothing ended up in the cast."
Kirsty

"We used sticker charts and rewards to help with eating issues."
Felicity

"Frozen yogurts were a staple for us."
April

Children are messy so always use a bib or cover the cast completely at meal times with a large shirt or apron.

"Our daughter was older and didn't want a bib so we got a couple of big t-shirts that she wore at meal times."
Felicity

"Our little one ate everything we did, just with an old dark shirt on."
Kirsty

"Get an apron or shirt for feeding so food doesn't go down the front of the cast."
Kris

In a similar vein, use beakers and cups with straws to avoid liquid spillages.

"We kept her water consumption up and found crazy straws to be very popular."
Susan

If you are breastfeeding your child there is no need to stop. You might need to try out different positions to ensure you are both comfortable but otherwise continue as you were.

Jenny Tschiesche (BSc Hons, Dip(ION) FdSc BANT), a leading nutrition expert, has provided the following simple post-operation diet advice (subject to allergies):

Addressing loss of appetite

Don't worry too much if your child has short-term loss of appetite following surgery. Focus on food quality and not quantity and, if age appropriate, let them to decide what they would like to eat – going for healthy options of course. If this continues and becomes a real concern speak to your GP.

Healing and rebuilding strength

Muscle tissue can be moved or damaged during surgery and the body needs protein to repair this. Making poultry, fish, eggs, natural yogurt, cheese, beans and nuts part of your child's diet will help this process.

High protein snacks such as peanut butter crackers, granola, natural yogurt with honey, nuts and cheese are a good idea.

Getting the right vitamins is vital for healing and both vitamin C and E are key players:

- Citrus fruits, strawberries, kiwi, peppers, Brussels sprouts, and broccoli are stacked with vitamin C
- Vitamin E rich sources include almonds, sunflower seeds, peanuts and avocado

Easy to digest foods

During your child's recovery you may find it easier to stick to a diet low in indigestible sugars, known as 'Low FODMAPS'. This is an acronym short for Fermentable Oligo-saccharides, Di-saccharides, Mono-saccharides and Polyols, which represents a select group of carbohydrates. These particular carbohydrates are poorly absorbed in the small intestine and are rapidly fermented by bacteria in the gut. This bacteria can cause tummy pain and problems with digestion.

High FODMAPS	Low FODMAPS
Fruit Apple, mango, watermelon, apricot, peach, plum	*Fruit* Banana, berries, citrus fruits, melon
Vegetables Asparagus, beetroot, broccoli, cauliflower, mushrooms, Brussels sprouts, cabbage, garlic, onions and leeks	*Vegetables* Sweet potato, parsnip, carrot, ginger, celery, swede, courgette, aubergine and tomato
Grains Wheat and rye	*Grains* Rice, oats, polenta, quinoa, millet
Dairy Milk, ice-cream, custard, soft unripened cheeses	*Dairy* Dairy-free milks, hard cheeses
Legumes Chick peas, haricot beans, kidney beans, lentils	

Constipation

Constipation can occur when a child is in a cast which isn't much fun for anyone, especially your child. Meat, wheat-based foods, refined and sugary foods as well as cheese and eggs can cause constipation so steer away for these and go for lots of vegetables, some fruit and lots of water.

Oat fibre can help prevent constipation and foods like ground flaxseeds are a mild laxative. If you feel constipation is a problem then do speak to your GP.

Avoiding nappy disasters

When your child is in a cast, you want their stools to be soft enough to eliminate easily but solid enough not to cause mayhem. Limiting processed sugar, eating Low FODMAPS foods (see above) and drinking sufficient water will all help keep things running smoothly.

A word of caution: foods like broccoli and apples can cause excess gas and wind so go easy on these. A dose of age appropriate probiotics can also be a good idea.

Chapter 9: Family and relationships

There is no point in sugar coating things: having a child with DDH can be draining and difficult for parents. Relationships and family dynamics can be put to the test, schedules thrown into disarray and plans changed at the drop of a hat but you will find a way to make it work.

Dr. Amanda Gummer, Research Psychologist Specialising in Child Development, commented, "Having a child with DDH can be a testing time for families. Parents feel stressed and pressed for time; siblings may feel anxious, guilty or left out and of course the child with DDH will be going through treatment.

"There's a tendency to assume that a condition such as DDH will be negative for a family. Whilst there can be added pressure and stress, this kind of experience can show you just how resilient you are and as the saying goes 'what doesn't kill you makes you stronger' and that is very much the case here.

"It is important that whatever you are dealing with and however many hurdles come along, you are all working towards a common goal of healthy hips for your child and that you do this together as a family."

How DDH affects you

In many cases, mothers are the main carers for a child when they are ill and this is no different for DDH, although not always the case. For both mothers and fathers, your instincts will kick in as you simply want to do the best for your child and make them better as soon as you can.

Everyone deals with the situation in different ways. Some find it an overwhelming trauma; others dig deep and find the positives. There is no right or wrong here, it's just what it is and you do what is best for you and your child.

Whilst I struggled with our DDH journey, looking at it now, it actually set me on a path to raise awareness and is the reason for this book. So for me the silver lining of a very difficult time is that my son is on the road to having healthy hips and there is more information to help parents like you.

"Yes DDH changed me and it's also driven me to set up my own business (www.hip-pose.co.uk) to help other parents."
Sam

"My daughter was seven when she was finally diagnosed and my heart breaks for her and all the things she's missing out on."
Joely

"DDH has made me stronger."
Kerry

"It's normal to get sad and frustrated but you will get over it quickly because your child needs you to be strong."
Colleen

"I have learnt to live with the now, as you don't know what will happen in the future and there is no point in thinking 'what if' all the time."
Gemma

"It's going to be hard. It's going to be really hard. It's not a journey anyone would choose. But everyone will be stronger and better for having taken it."
Heather

"Do not underestimate how strong, brave and resilient your child is. They will cope with it better than you could ever imagine."
Carol Anne

"In some ways, I was grateful for the diagnosis as it let me relax and go with the flow when it comes to parenting and I got closer to my daughter. Cuddling her to sleep instead of stressing over getting her to self-settle. As I discovered they learn how to do that all by themselves anyway, without sleep training, so thank you hip dysplasia for that!"
Anon

"It's left me in a horrible unknown place, anxious about the future...when you allow yourself to stop and think...it has taught us how resilient we can all be and to be thankful as much as possible for everything."
Melissa

"I cut my hours at work significantly, even though we needed the money, and it was the best thing I've ever done. She is my everything and DDH made us even closer."
Patricia

"Aside from regular everyday parenting and discipline, DDH made me ensure my child was surrounded with positive energy, kind and loving words, and most importantly encouragement."
Amanda

"I live in fear that she's not healing as well as she should and they'll tell me at her next visit that they'll have to operate again."
Gemma

Looking after yourself

I know you are amazing but you are not Wonder Woman or Super Man. It's really important to take each day as it comes. Forget about long term planning and thinking 'what if?' and 'why me?' and focus on the here and now.

DDH can take away feelings of control but you can get some of this back by maintaining routine. Whilst in the early days you might want to hide away, having structure and carrying on with life will retain a sense of normality. If you can do this then hospital trips, appointments and casts will become a part of that routine rather than the focus of your life.

You need to be in the best position mentally and physically so you can deal with DDH as well as the rest of your life. Be kind to yourself, you are doing the best you can.

"Take a time out when it's offered. YOU need it!"
Louise

"Don't have any major expectations, just take it day by day."
Melissa

"Don't hide away, do as much as you did before if you can. Yes you have to make adaptions but it's important for both you and your little one."
Jasmine

"It is a very stressful, and painful, time in one's family dealing with any illness, but that said, parents play a crucial part and need to be healthy to be able to help their children."
Patricia

"The amount of people who have said that it's gone quickly really have no idea what it is like. They don't

know you count down each day or that there's something you need to overcome to get a job done all the
time. You're constantly adapting things, and thinking of
how to keep a 14 month old entertained. It's hard and
emotionally draining but I know it will be worth it in
the long run."
Jaz

These sound obvious, but keeping things normal include simple
things such as:
- Build a support network you can rely on to help ease your
  load and give you some headspace. If you need help, ask
- Eat a well-balanced diet full of fresh fruit and vegetables,
  protein and good fat to keep up your strength and protect
  your immune system
- Take some exercise. Whether it's walking the dog, a bike
  ride or Zumba class, it will clear your head and the endor-
  phins released will make you feel brighter
- Keep up your hobbies and interests and don't let DDH become your life. You will find that even sitting down with a
  magazine and a cup of tea can be helpful
- Write a journal or start a blog. These can both be amazingly
  cathartic as well as a reminder of what a fantastic job you
  are doing and how far you have come. A great book to help
  with this is 'Blogging for happiness: a guide to improving
  positive mental health (and wealth) from your blog' by Ellen
  Arnison
- Enjoy a hot bath and an early night or even better, have a
  night off. Organise a trusted babysitter and take time out to
  relax and reconnect with your partner

Don't feel guilty if you take some time for you because in the
long run, doing so will help both you and your child. Eve
Menezes Cunningham, Holistic Therapist at the Feel Better
Every Day Consultancy, said, "It may sound like the most self-
indulgent thing in the world but self-care is KEY. The calmer

133

and more relaxed you can be, the better off your child will be, plus the rest of your family and others you come into contact with. This is not to beat yourself up on those natural occasions when you feel anything but calm, but to aim for feeling as good as possible yourself.

"Take a moment to think about a time when you felt completely at ease. It may be a memory from your childhood, more recent or even something you IMAGINE would feel peaceful. Take time to give your body a rest from current stresses by taking a mini mental holiday.

"Recount all the details from this moment - where you were, who you were with, how you felt, physical sensations, sounds, what you could see, any smells or tastes... If anything involved in this memory is currently a sad thought, change it. It needs to be an instant pick me up. Notice how you feel as you stay in your everyday life but just imagine this moment.

"We're all human and there'll be days when this feels impossible but notice the things that help you feel calm, relaxed, strong, happy and centred and make time for them however you can."

Your relationship with your partner

Whatever the severity of your child's DDH and however long their treatment takes, there will potentially be an impact on you and your partner. You may have lows, especially in the early days following the diagnosis and after treatments, and it will take time for you both to adjust as individuals and as a couple. Again, there's no right or wrong way to do this but the key to success is to communicate and be there for each other as well as giving one another space.

Dr. Amanda Gummer, added, "DDH can put immense pressure on a couple as they work together to deal with the issues a diagnosis throws up. However strong you are there will be times when anger, frustration, guilt, exhaustion, and sadness will bubble over and test even the strongest relationship.

"Whilst it might feel as if there is no end in sight with a plethora of appointments, scans and weeks in casts, if you can set up the right channels of communication and agree a plan of how to manage this period in your lives, you will be able to find positives.

"Blame and guilt might be felt but they are both wasted emotions so let go of them. Try to be honest with each other about how you feel, listen to each other and respect each other's feelings even if you don't agree with them."

"This journey that has taught my husband and I a lot about ourselves and has given us reason to love our daughter even more."
Anon

"I think that the whole experience made me and my husband stronger, we found that we complemented each other perfectly, where I was weak he was strong and vice versa. We pretty much realised that if we could survive this we could survive anything."
Laura

"DDH has made life tougher and affected my mental health, but we work as a team to do our best for our son."
Kirsty

"My husband and I took turns in taking my son out to give each other alone time, which really helped."
Anon

Oliver and I were both working for ourselves when we were going through this so we would try to go out for coffee together once a week. This would get us away from things, allow us to have some time together and it was a massive help. It wasn't an easy period in our marriage but each anniversary we now cele-brate makes me so proud of what we have achieved and proves how strong we are as a couple and family unit.

I think that it is important to mention the vital role of dads at this point. Mums do tend to take on the bulk of care for a child when they have DDH but this doesn't mean dads don't have a role to play and aren't affected by what is happening to their child.

They might not cry like we do or open up to family and friends with the same ease, but they still have to watch their child go through various procedures and pain.

For some, they will discuss their feelings but for many life goes on, something is broken and it will get fixed and maybe this is simply because facing the reality of the situation and watching their family suffer is all too much.

"My partner basically refused to really talk about our daughter's DDH because he said it was too hard and he didn't want to think about it. It was so hard not to have anyone to talk to who understood what was going on."
Amy

"I felt excluded from the whole process. From a point of view that hospital visits and ops and everything is centered around mums. Sounds weird but everyone ad-dressed my wife and I felt it was all 'mum this' and 'mum that' and it made me feel as if I wasn't included when I actually wanted to be."
Grant

"My dad says people forgot him, not once did they ask how he was feeling, it was all about him being strong for my mum and me yet in a funny way he needed more support. He was the one who carried me down to thea-tre and watched me be put under and then had to go

home and leave me there and also go to work. I think he was traumatised by it all."
Michelle

"As well as watching my son going through operations and months in casts I also had to keep it together for my wife and other child. DDH isn't easy but it is one of those things life throws at you and you have to get on with it until things get better. I look at my son now and am just so proud of how far he has come and I tend not to think about the past."
Oliver

"After the operation, my husband was the one who wasn't coping. He'd clammed up; I could see the pain in his eyes. He then lifted the blanket and there it was this huge white, damp cast bigger than what we expected. She looked engulfed by it. It was horrible."
Jaz

Keeping family and siblings strong

When siblings are added into the DDH mix you may feel as if you are being pulled in 101 directions, but it is vital that they aren't forgotten, feel included and loved.

There is so much going on and so much attention on the child with DDH that brothers and sisters can feel alone, left out and even guilty that it isn't them who needs treatment.

Whatever is going on, it is really important that your other children are part of the equation and that you take time to explain to them what is happening.

"DDH has given us as much hope as it has taken and shown us how strong we are as a family, how brave we can be and how much we can rise to a challenge."
Melissa

"It's been a very long process, and she still has more to come. We're very solid as a family, we've been through some very hard times and are good at supporting each other."
Sandra

"Many days are lost dealing with DDH. Although families evolve and cope, it feels like we missed out on some of the family time that we gave up. Marriages and siblings feel the effects of this too."
Alana

"My brother had dodgy legs when he was a baby but we fixed them and now he is better and I really love running with him in the garden."
Eddie

"DDH makes a family stronger and there is a light at the end of the tunnel."
Jo

"We had paper handmade snowflakes on the lounge room wall as a count down to cast off. We focused on one day at a time. If we had a bad day it was put behind us as we took a snowflake down."
Samantha

Dr. Amanda Gummer, further comments, "Just as you will have mixed feelings caused by your child's DDH, so will any siblings involved. They may feel angry, guilty, jealous, lonely or sad and it is your job to let them know this OK, it is normal and they are not to feel bad about thinking like this.

"The fact of the matter is, when a family is rocked by illness, siblings often don't get enough time with their parent and they can feel jealous and even resentful. It isn't easy but try not to favour the child with DDH and always side with that child as it can cause additional issues. What is really important is that you keep things fair, spend time with them each day so they feel loved and cared for too and keep an eye on any changes in behaviour and increased anxiety."

Top tips for family life whilst on your DDH journey include:

- Keep to existing family routines such as waking up times, mealtimes at the table, bed and bath times and regular activities as much as you can. There will be days when this simply isn't possible but the more you can keep to a routine the more settled everyone will feel as they will know what is coming next
- Be honest and communicate and try not to diminish children's concerns, frustrations or worries
- Ensure siblings understand they were not the cause of the illness and don't assume they don't blame themselves
- Schedule visits to see their brother or sister in the hospital if appropriate and possible
- If you are going into hospital with your child, ensure siblings know what is happening (depending on their age), when you will be back and who will be looking after them whilst you are gone
- Involve them in their brother or sister's after care if age appropriate
- Keep school or nursery up to date with the situation so they can look out for behaviour changes or issues in siblings. Being quiet and withdrawn or 'acting up' can indicate that they are feeling left out or worried and need some TLC and reassurance

Family and friends

It isn't unusual for friends and family members to be uncomfortable and unsure about how to respond to the news that your child has DDH. They could be worried, upset and shocked.

Close relatives and carers may, just like you, need time to adjust to the changes and emotions so give them the space they need. Involve them in important decisions about your child's care and treatment as appropriate and ask them for help if you need it – it can help them feel useful and valued.

"My family is much closer now as a result of the DDH. My parents helped us a lot, and so did all of our friends."
Anon

"Reach out for help, use your family, friends, professional help, and Facebook groups and forums."
Patricia

"As a family we will meet whatever is to come and for that we can say thank you to DDH as before we met you I had no idea we could take this on and how much strength my perfect little girl had to laugh her way through the majority of your visit."
Melissa

"Well my other daughter is 21 and she has been a strong supporter for me."
Joely

"Friends & family have been great!"
Bridgette

Well-meaning friends and family members may offer you advice about how to handle your child's treatment and readily compare DDH with illnesses they consider as being more serious.

"People would say 'be glad it's just this and not cancer' and that was not a good thing to say. Having a group of people to talk to and encourage each other is what matters most."
Karli

"Most family members thought DDH was no big deal, that the cast didn't look that hard to care for but ask for help and it was too much for them."
Colleen

"Sadly I fell out with my Mother-in-Law who visited us during my child's treatment (still unresolved). This was down to our stress levels which were at an all-time high."
Anon

"When my child's hip dislocated on Christmas morning, my Mother-in-Law said, 'Christmas is ruined'. I don't think I've ever been more disgusted at someone in my life."
Anon

This might be hard to handle and it can be easy to enter into disagreements and take umbrage because you are feeling emotional and vulnerable.

Rather than enter heated discussions, let them know you are making the best of the situation and following the advice of professionals. Don't let people's comments stop you taking your child out and about. You need to keep life as normal as possible and if you stay at home, away from human company you will probably feel even more lonely and isolated.

"Don't hide away, do as much as you did before if you can. Yes, you have to make adaptions, but it's important for both you and your little one."
Jasmine

Your child is as special and beautiful as any other child so do not be ashamed, do not take on other people's prejudices and if all else fails buy a lovely blanket and pop it over their spica, smile and carry on with your life.

Chapter 10: Life post cast

For many parents, cast removal day is the light at the end of the DDH tunnel. It's the prize you have been waiting for, the freedom your child craves and spells the end of the spica era.

That intense feeling of needing to hold your child cast free and hug them like your life depends on it is overwhelming and you just want to reach that point as quickly as possible. Anticipation, relief, thankfulness and normality are all part of that mixed bag of emotions.

Both times Lucas was taken out of his cast I cried with relief as I held him tight and was so glad I got him and his little body back.

"The first time round we felt relieved as we had 'made it' but she had to wear another cast and the second time we were more aware of what to expect and we were more realistic."
Felicity

"The spica coming off was a strange experience because we had been looking forward to 'that' day for so long and it was actually quite traumatic and surreal."
Amy

"After her first cast change one of her knees was free and it was the most beautiful day. We have the cast on for a while longer but this little bit of freedom showed us there is light at the end of the tunnel."
Patricia

"Cast off day and the weeks after were the best and the worst for us. We were so used to the cast protecting her, when it came off we were worried about her delicate

legs and the fear of walking, toilet training etc. At the same time it signaled the end of a long arduous journey, so it was well and truly worth it."
Grant

"Cast life just becomes the new normal. We almost missed it when it was taken off as it became part of our son."
Leah

"When they ripped the cast open she just looked so tiny and withered. The nurse told me I could pick her up and I panicked because I forgot how to hold her without the cast and I was scared I was going to hurt her."
Amy

Whilst having your child's cast taken off is a massive milestone, it is important to manage expectations and be realistic about what you might face. It might sound crazy but just as it takes time for a child to adjust to being in a cast, it can take time for them to adapt to being spica free.

This is yet another big change for them and as well as potentially being traumatised by the cast removal process, they might feel exposed and vulnerable without the security of a spica. Give it time, let them go at their own pace, encourage and praise them and ensure they feel safe and loved.

Cast removal process

As with pretty much everything DDH related, every case is different, so the amount of time your child will spend in a cast depends on their age, condition, surgery and surgeon.

When the spica cast is removed this is generally done in a plaster room/theatre without a general anaesthetic, but sometimes a child will need to be asleep. Your surgeon will let you know what will happen to your child so you can be prepared but try not to worry, you have done the hard work by this point.

If the cast is removed in the plaster theatre it will be done either using an electric saw or, as in our case, large scissors. The saw works by vibrations so it cannot cut the skin but it is noisy and may frighten your child and make you both nervous. Ensure you work with the medical team and let your child know that it will not hurt and you will be with them all the way through.

Staff will work as quickly as possible to get the spica off but it is a good idea to have something to keep your child occupied. A smart phone with a game for them to play or music to listen to, dummy, favourite teddy or blanket to keep them comforted and reassured can all help.

Once the cast is off, your child will have another X-ray to assess the position of the hip and success of the surgery. You should see your surgeon or a member of their team that day to discuss the X-ray results and make plans moving forwards.

Whatever the outcome of those X-rays, you have done an amazing job and deserve a massive pat on the back. I know this has been hard for you at times, but be proud of how far you have come and remember just what you have done for your child; given them a life with healthy hips.

Metalwork

If your child's had surgery that involved metal work (plates or screws) being placed in their hips, these will be removed under a general anaesthetic. Again, the amount of time they spend in hospital and the recovery period will depend on the child and your surgeon will give you the details.

Post-cast care

Once you are back at home you can start the next journey as a family but there are a few little things that might help make the transition smoother.

Once your child is cast free, you can pick them up as normal (they will feel really lovely and light) but it is advised that you still support their bottoms and hips. You will be surprised how you will do this out of habit and instinct anyway.

Do not expect your little one to stand up and run straight away, they probably won't. After spending weeks, even months, set in stone it is going to take time for them to get used to life without a cast and returning to normal may not be instant.

It is likely their little body will be stiff, less flexible and there may be some muscle tone loss. Give them the time and support they need to build their confidence and strength, it will happen.

"DDH doesn't end once the cast comes off. It's a case of learning to crawl and walk again. Using all the muscles that haven't been used for a while and you watch them gradually get stronger."
Felicity

"Many people seem to assume that once the socket is fixed that the DDH has been resolved, yet for many parents the fear doesn't go away. I think about DDH every single day and worry what the future will bring."
Emma

Skincare
Once their little legs are free, you will see a build-up of dry, flaky skin that might be discoloured, sore and scaly. Don't panic, this is perfectly normal but do be gentle with these areas as they will be sensitive.

Don't go for the soap and scrubbing brush straight away but instead start with tepid water and a soft cloth or flannel. Once they are happy with this, use a mild soap (organic, child specific are the best) and a gentle moisturiser on a daily basis and the dead skin will fall off in time and smooth legs will appear.

In older children you may also notice more hair than usual, but again in the weeks following their cast being removed this will fall out and the skin will repair itself.

Bath time
You might think that the first thing your child will want to do when they get home is have a bath as it was one of the daily

things they missed during those cast-clad days. Be prepared, a magical reunion might not be the case.

Before Lucas went into a cast he loved bath time but post-spica he was distressed and terrified which was quite a shock for us. He was the same with swimming so this was an unexpected issue to address and even now he is still pretty nervous of these situations.

If this does happen, go slow, let your child take the lead and in time they will get used to the water again and enjoy splashing around. They have been through a lot and there will be things they find scary, so you will need to do a lot of handholding and loving for a while, but that's all part of the fun.

Physical catch-up

Time spent in the cast may have helped create healthy hips but it can put physical development and skills on the back burner. We didn't receive any physio for Lucas and were told he would do things in his own time. Bouncing on trampolines and jumping out of trees wasn't allowed but letting him go at his own pace was key to his recovery.

I followed our surgeon's instructions about Lucas' return to physical activity and he did things when he was ready. This was much to the irritation of our Health Visitor who was obsessed with generic 'red book' milestones. She simply didn't seem to understand the implications of his DDH and the treatment he'd been through. I would become frustrated that despite reading his notes and me telling her he'd spent months and months in a spica cast, she was concerned he wasn't crawling, walking or stacking bricks like other children. It doesn't always happen like that for DDH kids.

"We had delayed walking but every other milestone was hit on target."
Elaine

"There was gross motor delay as well as delayed crawling and walking."
Anon

"She has missed out on school and dance and all things she should be doing. I hate seeing her feel lonely because friends abandoned her."
Joely

"During the second cast, our son stopped talking altogether, as we drove home from the hospital he said 'mummy'."
Oliver

"We are currently six months out of cast and she is walking and running but her muscles are still noticeably weak and she is unable to do certain things without help."
Felicity

"Two years post spica and Erin still has leg aches and struggles with her gross motor skills like riding a bike and running."
Emma

Jenny Seggie, Extended Scope Physiotherapist, commented: "For the majority of children, physiotherapy is not required once the plaster is removed, as they will gradually start to move around once they become more confident in their new freedom.

"In some cases though, especially when an older child requires surgery, physiotherapy can be helpful to build the child's confidence in movement so they are moving without even realising it. Formal exercise programmes often aren't required and I have found that simply playing in water can be extremely beneficial. The act of getting in and out of the pool, even if shuffling on their bottom, gives them independence and once in the water floats and toys can be used to encourage the child to move through the water in order to chase them.

"For a child who is more confident in water, games that encourage weight bearing, such as walking races can be encouraged to work on their range of movement by asking them to race forwards, backwards or sideways. I have also added flippers on occasion to add more resistance and exaggerate their movements.

"At home, you can play games with small gym balls or 'space hoppers'. They can be encouraged to sit on them with their feet on the floor and play 'Simon Says'. Encouraging them to move their arms will change the pressure they put through their lower limbs and rolling their bottoms forwards and backwards will flex their hips.

"Fun is definitely the key to encouraging a frightened child to move around, so use any activity your child finds fun and non-threatening and let your imagination run wild. If in doubt please contact your local Paediatric Physiotherapy Team and they will be able to advise you on what is safe for your child."

Do not worry though. You have been through the hardest bit, they will 'catch up' and you can enjoy watching them do this. In time they will start to move again, gradually gain confidence and pick up where they left off.

Letting go

Whilst it is natural to want to keep your child safe after all they have been through, it is important to look beyond DDH and see a little boy or girl who needs, and wants, to be like everyone else.

I won't lie, this can be a challenge but having worked so hard for those healthy hips you need to try to let go and let them spread their wings.

> "My son is 4.5 months post spica and I am literally terrified of playgrounds, but at the same time he is desperate to play and fit in!"
> *Fiona*

"How can you stop them trying to be 'normal' children? As a DDH mum you have to adjust some things and let her try."
Felicity

"It's only natural to be afraid for our children because they do not see the potential hazards we do. I still worry at almost two years post-op."
Simonne

"I avoided a lot of things because I had PTSD and it was too stressful for me to put her in the position where she might fall and hurt herself."
Jen

"Trampolines are my fear but we have no restrictions and I have to just let her be a normal kid."
Leanne

"When she's messing about with her sisters, they pull each other about I find myself saying 'mind her legs'."
Anon

"Trampolines!! That would be the death of me."
Fiona

"One year post spica with no restrictions from our surgeon and I still won't let my daughter jump in a bouncy castle with other children. I am unreasonably sensitive but try to keep this inside so I don't give her the impression she is fragile. But wow, it is hard!"
Susan

"I try not to be cautious but when it's icy and cold it's hard not to be."
Felicity

Dr. Rachel Andrew, BPS Associate Fellow & HCPC Registered Clinical Psychologist, said, "When a child goes through the riggers of DDH treatment, your instinct is to love and protect them. Once they are cast free and recovering, they need childhood normality to return and parents need to try to let go. These kids are tough and need to be allowed to become their own person not a shadow of their condition.

"This can be hard but you worked so hard to get hips healthy, let them be used. Of course listen to your surgeon when it comes to what they can and cannot do, but apart from that see your child aside from their DDH and carry on with life.

"In the main, if they want to go the park, splash around in the pool or play football, let them do it. It might take a while for you to feel OK about this but let's face it you wouldn't be the parent you are if you didn't feel this way. Be sensible, but don't wrap them up in cotton wool and define them by DDH. They've spent long enough living with restrictions and extreme boundaries, now they need to fly."

There are some DDH cases where there will be other conditions such as hyper mobility and leg-length discrepancies and these will be identified by your medical team and assessed as necessary.

We have to remember that these kids are fighters and are blessed with the spirit needed to deal with the challenges thrown at them. If they can do it, so can you.

Emotional catch up

You will be able to see the physical progress your child is making day-by-day, but when their cast is taken off a magic wand isn't waved to make everything inside ok and that can be tricky.

Dr. Rachel Andrew, further commented, "Just because your child's cast has been taken off and the physical wounds are fading, the emotional scars can take longer to heal. Recovering from traumatic experiences can take time; your child will go at their own pace and deal with things as best they can. Some children become more aggressive and have meltdowns, others may become withdrawn, there isn't a one size fits all reaction. Whilst it is impossible to fully understand what they are going though, you can help them deal with this.

"Don't rush them, be aware of their moods, be consistent with your reactions and over time things will hopefully improve. You will never know whether their behaviour is due to their DDH experiences or just part of their personality, therefore it is vital not to define them by their hips. By the same token, they're a normal child so don't let them off bad behaviour because of their treatment.

"If you aren't seeing progress and are concerned, talk to your GP or health visitor to explore further what is happening and how they can help move things forwards."

"My child suffered with sensory issues, almost a sort of PTSD. She also has noise issues and a fear of swings and being up high."
Karen

"She put on weight from not bring able to be active and is now going through PTSD and some eating issues. It has just been a lot all around on my girl."
Joely

"We haven't experienced anything terrible that I am aware of thank goodness but she is a little angrier than she used to be and we are working on this."
Laura

"My son is terrified of plasters so the drip was his worst part of the hospital. He is scared of nurses and fearful in certain situations, like going to the doctor."
Fiona

"My daughter suffered with anxiety, poor fine and gross motor skills (which are developing) and was a very fussy eater."
Felicity

"To even get our son to have his flu jab or a routine tooth check-up is a real battle and as for follow-up X-rays, it is a total nightmare."
Oliver

"She was a little reserved and didn't want to go back to school but started to warm up to the kids who were so helpful. She was a little sensitive after getting her cast off as well."
Anon

"Lacked confidence but that's improved."
Kelly

Whilst all of these need consideration, try not to let feelings of guilt stop you from maintaining clear boundaries for your child. Lashing out in anger and frustration might well be a part of what has happened to a child but at the same time, DDH cannot be used as an excuse for bad behaviour and if this isn't addressed you may have more problems moving forwards.

Eve Menezes Cunningham, Holistic Therapist and Founder of the Feel Better Every Day Consultancy commented: "Allow your child to feel whatever s/he is feeling and hold that space for them. Make the whole spectrum of emotions OK using safe, appropriate expressions of anger, hurt, sadness, loss and even joy.

"Encourage safe movement. Stamping feet can be grounding for both of you as well as making you laugh (and laughter's another great way to discharge stress). Stamping feet honours anger as well as that ancient fight/flight impulse. It can burn off a lot of the stress hormones in your system. Similarly, punching pillows gets it out so you can move forward. Notice what your child wants to do and if appropriate, support it."

As your child develops and begins to recover they will need to accept that everything does not revolve around them and this is certainly an issue we had with Lucas until he was five.

One of the key things for us was to find activities and toys he really enjoyed as well as encouraging him to play with his brother and friends. At home and at nursery we worked on him sharing and taking turns. We also had to ensure he knew he couldn't have his own way all the time, something he still struggles with now and again.

My advice would be to pick your battles, spend time with your child, watch how they play and relate to others, ensure they feel safe and secure and over time things should calm down and a new equilibrium will be found.

Follow-up appointments

The schedule of follow up appointments will once again depend on your child. Appointments are more regular when your child is younger and growing but as time goes by and things become stable, there will be longer between visits.

At each appointment your child will probably have an X-ray as this is the most effective way to see how the hip joint is developing and a catch-up meeting with your surgeon.

Remember, when you go to these appointments try to be as truthful about where you are going and why with your child (age appropriately of course). They might really hate hospitals but try to reassure them it's just to check everything is OK. Take things to keep them occupied whilst you are there and even give them a treat when you leave and this way it is manageable.

I have said it a lot but DDH is not a textbook condition, these kids are not textbook kids, they are strong children whose bodies and brains have had a lot to deal with and in time they will find their way.

It is easy to see other children the same age as yours steaming ahead, and compare your child with them, but don't. Day-by-day and step-by-step they will find their own way and be the best they can and that is far more than good enough in my book.

If there are any issues you are not happy with between appointments, speak to your surgeon and get some advice. It might be nothing but if it is, you will be glad you checked.

Take one day at a time. You and your child have worked hard to get where they are today and it will take them a bit of time to catch up.

Chapter 11: Lucas

Lucas is the reason why I wrote this book and this is our story:

After a relatively easy birth, Lucas was born at 04.38 on 13 June 2009 but a newborn check the next day showed a 'clicky' right hip. Little did we know that one small word, 'clicky', signaled that a long, hard journey was ahead of us.

Whilst clicky hips are not a diagnosis of DDH, alarm bells rang given the strong history of the condition in my family with my younger sister being diagnosed as a baby and a cousin still suffering. I raised this with the nurses and was told the details would be placed on his hospital notes before we were discharged and a scan appointment would be organised.

Neither happened.

The happiness of a new baby took over and it wasn't until Lucas' six-week check I remembered the clicky hip and told my GP as there weren't any details on the hospital notes. However, she didn't think there was a problem and neither did the Health Visitor when she visited around the same time.

However, DDH was now front of mind so I pushed for the scans my first son had been given because of the family history, and to this day I am so thankful I did.

Following another examination, a scan was offered to cover all eventualities. Over the coming weeks, Lucas seemed to be progressing well, trying to turn over and kicking his legs with no visible difficulties in moving, however from the way he would lie on me like a cat and the slight difference in the creases in his legs, I knew things weren't quite right.

The day of the scan eventually arrived and the sonographer told me in a very matter of fact way that my son had DDH and that they would be seeing a lot more of us in the future.

I was left crying in the darkened scanning room as my baby looked up at me with those innocent blue eyes. I would have done anything to take away the pain and suffering I knew he would have to endure in the coming weeks, months and years.

I was filled with anger, confusion and grief. I reverted to that scared little girl whose baby sister was stuck in traction and inside I was silently screaming 'why him, why me, why us?'

I was told that Lucas would need to wear a Pavlik harness for between 12 and 20 weeks and that this course of treatment would put his hip back in place. There was no handholding, no pleasantries or gentleness and this heartless treatment is something we will never forget and find hard to forgive.

The following day, my husband and I took Lucas back to the hospital where he was placed in the harness and went from being placid and content to miserable and fretful. It was clear that the harness wasn't only uncomfortable but that it was causing him anguish and discomfort. He didn't want to feed or sleep, the constant crying was intolerable and I felt helpless.

I spent hours scouring the Internet for information but all I found was a host of horror stories, out of date statistics and images of archaic contraptions. I sat with tears streaming down my face as I read story after story of suffering, splints, trauma and divorce. I turned off the laptop and battled through with the support of my husband, who was amazing, and close family, wishing there was just one book I could buy and take comfort from.

As the days passed, Lucas was restless and unhappy, not sleeping and obviously distressed. I called the nurse to check whether this was normal and was treated like the neurotic mother I was obviously perceived to be. She told me to give him Calpol and that he would get used to the harness just as he would a new pair of dungarees from Mothercare. Nice.

This was the first time, but far from the last, I was expected to treat DDH like a minor issue: a blip, a cut finger that you simply cover up and get on with.

Ten days later we were told that Lucas' hip was now in the right position and that all we could do now was sit it out and wait for nature to take its course and the harness was to stay on.

But something didn't fit. My mothering instincts kicked in once again and I simply wasn't going to sit around and do nothing and watching my son being miserable if it wasn't necessary.

I did a little more research and soon realised that four and a half months was pretty late for my baby to be put in a Pavlik harness and to remain in it for up to 20 weeks was ridiculous. My husband agreed and we sought a second opinion and thank goodness we did.

After an X-ray, we were told that Lucas had Tonnis Grade 3 acetabula dysplasia with subluxation on his right hip and only surgery would correct the problem.

Finally we had someone who knew what they were doing and could help Lucas. All we ever wanted was for our baby to be healthy and happy and now there was a glimmer of hope that this could be the case again.

Christmas came and went in a blur and in February 2010, at just eight months old, Lucas was admitted for a closed reduction, the first of many operations.

Handing over my baby to the medical team was one of the hardest things I have had to do as a mother. My husband said he would take him but I felt it was my job and as much as it hurt, I wanted to be there for him. They wheeled Lucas away from me and then bought him back several hours later in a frog plaster that was twice, if not three times, the weight of him.

I can't thank my husband enough for his support as Lucas came round in pain and groggy from the anesthetic and disorientated by his new 'trousers'. There he was, blond-haired and blue eyed, incarcerated in heavy plaster with just a hole for his nappy and whilst he should have been wearing cute jeans, all that would fit were leg warmers and vests – cute maybe, heart-breaking certainly.

The staff were kind and showed us both how to roll him over, lift him, change him and together we worked out the best ways for him to fit into his buggy and the new car seat we had bought for this day.

The operation was done, the cast was set and life went on back at home. We kept things as normal as we could. We moved house, I set up a new business, we went to the park, took Eddie (Lucas' older brother) to nursery and even went on holiday. But I won't lie, it was very hard. As well as having to care for Lucas, Eddie needed my attention, care and love and so did my husband who was going through this too. My husband was always very level headed: it was broken and we would get it fixed and if it hadn't been for his approach and calm manner I don't know how I would have coped. I know there were times when it was too much for him and that seeing his son in the cast was tough but he knew it was for the best and the only way Lucas would ever get better.

Of course, at nine months most babies are trying to crawl and pull themselves up on the furniture and putting their feet on the floor but my baby couldn't do that. He coped amazing well and adapted to the situation. Eddie would play with him on the floor, bringing him puzzles and books to look at and sit with him watching TV on a massive beanbag.

Whilst Lucas amazed us with his bravery and strength, the looks, stares and comments from strangers would astonish and upset us even more.

There was the man in Boots who did a second take and then got his kids to come and look at the 'funny kid' in the buggy.

The woman and her friend in Zara for came for a second look at the 'special baby' and sniggered when I asked them if there was a problem.

The tin rattler in the High Street who asked me what I had done to him.

The Big Issue seller who looked at us with pity.

The friend who said "at least it isn't cancer".

These comments and actions made me angry and sad. They made me fiercely protective of both my sons and I was so thankful neither really understood what was happening or how others were reacting.

The looks and comments made me cry. They made me anxious and depressed. However, looking back, they made me stronger and made me fight for the hips my son deserved.

There were arguments and dark moments but we got on with life and after four months Lucas came out of the cast and was placed into a softer harness that could come off for an hour a day.

This offered a little respite because not only was it lighter and Lucas could pull himself around and he was given one hour of freedom a day when he could explore, have a bath, enjoy cuddles and be free once again. Three months later he was let loose a little more, wearing the harness only at nap times and night, which meant he could enjoy his first birthday, a great day with the family and friends who had supported us so much, cake and presents as well as smiles and hope for us.

At the end of July we were thrilled to be told that the closed reduction had worked, the ball and socket were sitting neatly in place and we had to now give Lucas' body time to grow and heal.

My husband and I celebrated with champagne that night and watched with pride, and relief, as they played together as brothers should do. Lucas was able to go back into his normal clothes, enjoy his toys once again and sleep in his cot without a cast knocking against the bars and keeping him awake.

Whilst he was a little more frustrated than the placid baby who went into the cast, our toddler was enjoying life once again and his smile would light up the room. I knew he was a heartbreaker in the making but little did I know it was our hearts that were going to break before any pretty teenage girl's.

As the months went by, Eddie started school and Lucas and I would spend time together building his strength, going to soft play classes and making up for the lost months he spent in a cast.

His leg lengths were fine, the creases were now matching, he was expert crawler and could pull himself up on furniture but I had a nagging feeling that he wasn't as strong as he should be and progress was slower than I had expected.

I called the hospital and at an earlier than scheduled appointment our world crumbled again. We were told that Lucas' hip wasn't forming as they had hoped and they were going to have to start surgery again. He was booked in for an open reduction and a femoral osteotomy in June and hysterical is the only word I can use to describe my reaction.

I was broken. I didn't think I could do it again. I didn't want him to suffer again. I didn't want him to have metal bolts in his hip. I didn't want his leg to be broken and repositioned. I didn't want him to spend another six months in a cast from his chest to his ankles with a stick between his legs. I didn't want people staring at him again. I didn't want to have to ask my family and friends for help and support. I didn't want Eddie to have to be second best again. I didn't want my marriage to be put under pressure again.

I DIDN'T WANT THIS.

The thing was, we didn't have any choice. Lucas had to have the surgery but I just wished we didn't have to go through it all over again.

Life went on, the boys played together, Lucas was walking but with a pretty pronounced gait and my heart broke over and over again thinking about the future.

There was an outbreak of chicken pox locally and we decided to have the boys vaccinated because I couldn't imagine anything worse than to be stuck in a cast and covered in itchy, sore spots – that would be like adding insult to injury.

It's the little things like this that you have to think about when your child has DDH. You almost have to be able to second guess the future and plan for every eventuality. On one hand it makes you very organised and aware but on the other, it isn't quite how you imagined family life would be and you can become obsessed.

Spring came and went and after taking the holiday we had booked as a treat when we were originally told Lucas was in the clear, we started to plan for his next surgery.

We talked to him and his brother about needing to have another trip to fix his legs. Lucas was too young to really understand but Eddie had a lot of questions and was determined to help get his brother's 'dodgy legs' better.

The day of surgery arrived and I just wanted to get it over and done with and carry on with our lives and beat DDH.

The nursing staff were amazing and couldn't do enough to help us but I actually found round two more difficult than the first. He was second on the list that morning but we had taken lots of toys and the nurse gave him a pre-med which made him pretty chilled and happy to listen to Thomas stories and watch a DVD.

The walk down to theatre broke me. I didn't want to let go of his tiny, limp hand once he was under but I walked away knowing that we were one step closer to the finish line.

After several hours in theatre he was back in recovery and in a full body spica with a broomstick between his legs.

He picked up pretty quickly and after a loud night on the ward, we went home and life went on. I was on autopilot and worked out the best way to carry him, how to change his nappy (the hole was bigger this time) and the narrow spica meant he was able to fit into the buggies we had at home.

It is fair to say that over the nine weeks Lucas was in this spica he became increasingly angry and frustrated. He almost stopped talking, instead choosing to scream and grunt. He would smash his cast on the floor and his eyes lost the sparkle that had made them dance only weeks before. You can kind of understand this. One minute there he was walking (with a wobble) and playing and the next his independence had been taken away from him and he was stuck on the floor in those concrete pants and he was cross. I think I would have been too.

We did all we could to make him happy. We had a spica table, bean bags, two sets of wheels and for his birthday he got a ride-on tractor that worked with his cast – that did get a cheeky smile of approval. We would go to the park where he could fit in the swings and luckily it was a good summer and he loved to be in the garden with his brother.

Lucas was pretty good at getting about and by the time he was set free his upper body strength was impressive. There was no stopping him when it came to moving around in his cast but he wasn't happy, little things frustrated him and he closed down just a little more each day.

One of the worst days was when we went to the school fete at my older son's new school and Lucas was totally miserable, hot and very cross. He didn't want to be in the buggy, he didn't want to be on the floor or on my knee. The more noise he made the more people looked and more stressed we felt. I remember a lady asking if she could take him for a walk for me. I said no, it was my job, but that gesture has stayed with me and we have been friends ever since.

Strangers still stared. There was the odd tut and raised eyebrows from someone assuming his legs were broken because of something we did. I tried to let this go and was just thankful that he wouldn't remember any of it and it was my job to protect him from any ignorance he was exposed to. Those who did ask what was wrong often had experience of DDH themselves and were very sweet and concerned – that made a big difference.

Life went on. I worked, Lucas got stronger, we were getting Eddie ready to start school and we enjoyed watching the London Olympics on beanbags with popcorn. Each day was marked off on a sticker board and eventually we were in the car heading back to the hospital for the cast to come off.

By this point Lucas had a fear of the hospital and all medical staff. Getting the cast off was quite an ordeal and the follow-up X-ray was traumatic to say the least, as he didn't want anyone to touch him. He just wanted to be close to mummy and daddy.

The silver lining was that his hip was now in place, the open reduction and femoral osteotomy had been successful and we were free to go home.

There were tears of joy and relief, hugs and kisses. I had my boy back and on the way home he said "mummy" and I crumbled as it was the first time he had spoken properly for weeks.

This time round we did see progress and slowly but surely the anger died down but didn't totally disappear. I am not sure if he was depressed but Lucas certainly wasn't the little boy he could have been and was diagnosed with Post Traumatic Stress.

Having something tangible to work with gave us a focus rather than blaming things on the terrible twos (I am sure there was an element of this in the mix too) and in time we found ways to bring him out of himself.

As he slowly adjusted to a 'normal' life free of poking and prodding and with no casts or appointments in the calendar, he settled down and stopped living on a knife-edge of unpredictability and hospital visits.

Just as Lucas started to relax, so did we. Our life and relationship got back on track and whilst there is no doubt I lost a friend or two, I also realised just who mattered and who would be there for us through thick and thin.

A year on from that surgery, his metal work was removed, he started school and his anger started to subside. He has become Lucas, the little boy he was trying so hard to be and not the kid in a cast.

I had to start letting go and that is how this book came about. I couldn't keep feeling sad about the card we were dealt and needed to stop wrapping him up in cotton wool as it wasn't healthy. He needed to be able to go out and play with his friends, childhood memories are made in parks and on scooters and with so many opportunities already missed, this had to be made possible for him.

'Be careful' and 'stop' were well used phrases in our parenting vocabulary and as much as I wanted to protect the legs we had worked so hard to fix, if I didn't let him spread his wings and fly, what would have been the point?

He dances Gangnam style with his brother and sings at the top of his voice and watching him so happy and free is bitter sweet. X-rays at an annual check revealed that as a result of Lucas' femoral osteotomy, his legs aren't the same length. Whilst the difference isn't massive, it is big enough for everything to be out of kilter and he will need a pelvic osteotomy. This news floored me when we were told. I wasn't expecting it but we are determined not to fall apart and to get him, and all of us, through this.

DDH is not something I would have chosen but in a funny way it has made us stronger and shown me just what being a mother is all about: putting your child's needs (emotional and physical) above yours and loving unconditionally.

I love my boys and husband more than I ever thought possible and whilst DDH has revisited us, we are living and loving the life we have and take this new challenge one day at a time.

Chapter 12: Case studies

Erin

Erin was a third child and born at full term. There was no family history of DDH and although she was a big baby, 8lb 13ozs at 38 weeks gestation, she had none of the known birth markers associated with DDH.

Erin was a frequent visitor to the GP with repeated ear and chest infections. She had several hospital admissions for her chest and attended all her development checks but her DDH diagnosis was late.

At her nine-month check (she was actually 11 months) Erin's mum, Emma, voiced her concerns regarding Erin's mobility as she was sitting but not crawling or weight bearing. This was the first time Emma heard the words Developmental Hip Dysplasia. The Health Visitor noted that Erin's thigh creases were not symmetrical and Emma was reassured this would be monitored. Monitoring consisted of a few phone calls where Emma confirmed Erin was still not walking.

When Erin did take her first steps at nineteen months, her parents were immediately concerned that something was very wrong as she had an obvious limp and dragged her right leg. After an emergency GP appointment Erin was referred to physio who found that Erin was 'intoeing' a little but decided that it would correct itself with time. However, as Erin walked out of the appointment the physio spotted the limp and called them back in. She concluded that Erin had a leg length discrepancy and would need orthotics.

Emma was still unhappy and went back to her GP who examined Erin yet again. This time he said he could feel her hip crunching and referred them to a paediatrician who took one look at Erin limping and told Emma that he suspected DDH. Erin was sent straight to X-ray and a phone call the following morning confirmed that she had DDH and had been referred to orthopaedics. The shock at this late diagnosis was overwhelming and Emma thought back to the remarks that Erin would be monitored following her nine-month check.

Their appointment was two weeks later and the X-rays showed Erin's right hip socket was very shallow and underdeveloped. Erin was moved to the top of the operation list and was admitted to hospital just 12 days later for a closed reduction. The treatment plan was for a closed reduction followed by 18 weeks in a spica cast with cast changes at six and twelve weeks. Erin would then have a six to ten week break before having a Salters Osteotomy and a further six weeks in spica. The K Wires would then be removed when the cast was removed. This treatment involved six trips to theatre.

Although Erin coped very well, the experience has left her much weaker than her peers. She became subdued in spica and did not talk much. Being in a spica meant that she was not experiencing the world like her friends and this affected her development.

Looking after an older child in spica is physically demanding. Not only were additional car seats, buggies, seating arrangements and clothes needed but lifting and carrying Erin was hard and this took its toll on Emma who had to do the bulk of the care.

Erin is now two years post spica but still doesn't walk as far as her peers. The legacy of a late diagnosis means the family are waiting to see what further treatment could be necessary in the future.

Emma feels very angry that the DDH was missed and wishes Erin could have had the opportunity to try a Pavlik harness at an early age to see if her hips could have been fixed without surgery.

Emma has campaigned for more awareness of DDH and was a great help and inspiration for this book.

Sophie

Sophie was diagnosed with DDH at eight months when she had an unsuccessful closed reduction. This was followed by a successful open reduction at 17 months. After regular checks, Sophie was discharged at age nine and we thought that was the end of DDH for us.

When she was 13 she started to complain of pain and how her hip kept clicking, so I took her to our GP who sent her for an X-ray. Our new surgeon informed us she had developed AVN, a condition that is caused when the neck of the femur grows abnormally.

It was hard coping with a young child in a hip spica but having a teenager with hormones who is unable to get around has challenges too. We are now four weeks post AVA surgery, Sophie is on crutches, she is having intensive physio and is back at school part time.

Sophie still has a way to go and it will be two years before we know if the operation has been successful. She will need a hip replacement as an adult but hopefully her hip can be preserved for as long as possible. The main aim was for Sophie to become pain free and we are hoping that will happen soon.

Michele

The question is, do I have DDH or does DDH have me? I was born in 1975 and was a miserable baby from the start. I didn't like being cuddled, being in a pram or having a nappy changed, which in hindsight isn't surprising.

As I got older it became more obvious that there was something very wrong with my left hip. I'd always had an extra crease on my leg that no health professional could explain and when it came to walking, I not only had a limp but would also drag my leg behind me. My parents kept taking me to see our GP but they said I was miserable and lazy. How very wrong they were.

In the end, my Nana took me to see her GP who arranged for me to go to hospital the next day where X-rays confirmed I had DDH. They started treatment there and then.

I was placed on a wooden board attached to a cot and every day for six months they stretched my legs until they curled up under the back of my head in the hope it would put the hip joint back in place. This failed so I had an operation and then I was placed in a spica for three months. Sadly this also failed so the plan was to then break my hip and pelvis and pin it all back together and place me in another plaster cast for many months. I had to have this done twice.

"When I was seven, problems surfaced again and my metal work was removed. I had physio and walked with a frame for a few months afterwards but I then had to get on with life. I was really lucky until I hit my teenage years. When I was 14, the pain started to become bad but I muddled through on painkillers.

I went on to have two children and that has been my biggest challenge. I'm not the wife and mother I was and that makes me sad. I've slowed right down and I can't do as much as I want to do. I need help with my cleaning, I walk with crutches but needing a wheelchair and mobility scooter are edging closer and this scares the life out of me.

There were so many operations and so much pain that I had to give up my career as a nurse. This was heart breaking as I loved my work and making a difference to people's lives was amazing.

I've fought against DDH all my life and I will continue that fight no matter how hard or painful it is. I'm really frightened of what the future holds and how this will end but I know that while I have my amazing husband, children, family and friends I will be fine.

Lucy

My daughter, Lucy, was born full term but was very small and extended breech. When you see your newborn for the first time and their left leg is bent behind their head like a yogic master, you kind of expect there will be consequences but despite checking her, DDH was not detected.

At six weeks we took Lucy for a routine hip check and were upset, but perhaps not surprised, to discover that her left hip was dislocated. She weighed just over 6lbs at the time and had to be fitted with the smallest Pavlik harness they could find. I remember feeling numb and very protective of my tiny baby as this alien and constricting harness was put on her. The timing of the DDH diagnosis could not have been worse as just a few days before, we had learned that Lucy has a unique genetic fault on two of her chromosomes. Because it was unique, there was no evidence to what the future would hold apart from it being bleak in terms of her health and development.

The nurses who treated Lucy were very kind and helped me to focus on the DDH as something that was treatable and could be fixed. It was summer, so although it pained me to have to cut up all her lovely new clothes to fit over the harness, at least she would not be cold. I was instantly hit, however, like a truck in the face, when complete strangers would look at my daughter and gasp or make senseless comments. Luckily Lucy took to wearing a harness with ease, although it did make the colic a little more difficult as she couldn't lie on her front.

After six weeks of treatment the harness came off, the left hip had realigned and all looked normal, so it was devastating that at the six month checkup it was discovered that it had come out again. This time we were talking about surgery and she was still very little. A new team of people swept into our lives, to join the by now growing team of paediatricians and therapists helping with Lucy's medical and developmental needs.

I still feel genuinely lucky that the team treating Lucy's hip dysplasia were so fantastic. They treated me like an equal and wanted my opinions, they were humorous and yet extremely professional and most of all they doted over Lucy. It was decided that due to Lucy's slow growth, we would wait until she was a year old to do the surgery. As the date drew closer, I started to panic about coping when Lucy was in a hip spica cast. The difficult nappy changes, how to carry her, whether she would sleep, how we could get her into a car seat/push-chair/high chair. The list of complications to our already complex life seemed endless. I was signposted to a charity called STEPS who provide advice to parents on DDH and lower limb conditions. We bought a Britax two way elite car seat with special hip-spica adaptations, our Occupational Therapist obtained a hip-spica chair on loan and luckily the lovely pink pushchair I'd treated myself and Lucy to was an ok shape to take her in a cast.

The day of surgery arrived, and we anxiously waited in a room with another couple whose daughter was due the same procedure. The mum and I quickly made friends and to this day are very close as it turns out her daughter also has a rare chromosome condition and our girls are now best buddies in the same class at school. Having a friend going through the same DDH journey proved to be really helpful. Today there are many social media sites with groups dedicated to DDH and the mutual support parents give to each other is heartwarming and much needed.

I will never forget that first operation, as I soothed Lucy whilst she was anesthetised for the first time. Nothing prepares you for it, you just have to have faith and a lot of trust that the doctors know what they are doing. Overwhelmed with adrenaline, I spluttered out "Promise me she won't die" shortly followed by "Promise me you'll use the purple cast" luckily I said these in the right order! As crazy as it sounds, having a coloured cast seemed the only way to me to avoid the horrible comments I'd heard other mums face. One local mum had told me that on her first day out with her daughter in cast, she had been approached by a stranger who'd asked if she had dropped her child down the stairs! Now I know a full hip-spica cast can look a bit alarming, but really I was speechless when I heard this, and very angry.

It was now approaching winter with frequent rain (like gremlins the cast must not get wet we were warned!) so I designed and made a pair of waterproof trousers to fit over Lucy's cast. We still had many other medical and therapy appointments to get to plus I refused to keep her shut indoors for the three months of treatment. At one of her hip checkups, the nurse and surgeon both remarked on her trousers saying they had never seen anything like it before and how wonderful they were. I also noticed that when the trousers were on no one took a second glance at us; it was as if the cast was invisible. Encouraged, I made the trousers in a range of fabrics and actually had fun dressing my 'hip kid' as the months passed. They also came in useful after the cast was finally removed as Lucy's legs used to being held apart, stayed in that position for a couple of weeks. The hip-spica trousers allowed for her stretched ligaments to contract in their own time and not be forced into regular clothes.

At about this time, it had become clear that I would not be able to return to work as Lucy needed specialist care and her small army of therapists produced a grueling schedule for us. I can't say that giving up my career in museums was easy, I mourned for it for a long while. However, the surgeon and physiotherapist continued to say I had a great idea with the clothing. So I went back to the drawing board and created a specially designed sleep suit and a romper to be worn over a Pavilk harness. The hospital staff provided me with willing parents happy to trial the designs and I gave them a sleepsuit as thanks. I got their feedback and comments and one lady very kindly agreed to her daughter being the 'model' for Hip-Pose.

The creation of Hip-Pose was a whirlwind journey. I got a business mentor, registered as a Ltd company, won a £2,000 startup grant, sourced a manufacturer in the UK, designed my own website, got a logo, taught myself pattern making and finally went 'live' online all within a year of making that first pair of trousers for Lucy. If asked again, I really don't know where I got the energy from to stay up late night after night and to spend the few spare hours when Lucy was in nursery on the business. Looking back I realise now that this was my therapy, my way of pushing through the pain and grief of having a child with profound special needs. Everyone deals with the news differently and it felt imperative to me to create something positive out of a difficult situation. I had felt firsthand what it is like to feel embarrassed about your child's treatment aid and be wary of going into social situations only to be challenged by another rude comment. I felt, and still do feel, passionately about helping parents to go about their everyday life as normally as possible at a difficult time. Dressing your child should be a fun activity and providing a practical solution to the problem was my main aim.

I hope to eventually reach out to every DDH parent and tell them about Hip-Pose, how to survive this difficult time and come out of it a little less battle worn!

Daisy

Daisy was diagnosed with hip problems at her paediatric check-up when she was a day old. A scan a few days later showed she had a severe case of bilateral DDH. There was nothing holding the hip joints in place at all and I went into total shock.

They fitted Daisy with a Pavlik harness straight away. I had never heard about DDH before and was put in touch with STEPS for support. I was distraught, as we couldn't bathe her, she didn't go in her car seat and couldn't use the travel system that we had bought either.

The surgeon explained that the harness had to work for both hips, not just one, or she would need surgery. I had to take her back every week to have the harness adjusted and then she had a scan every other week.

When visiting the hospital one time someone had parked their car so close to mine that I couldn't get her back in the car. I just stood in the car park in tears until a kind lady came over to see if I was OK. She held Daisy in her pram so that I could pull the car forward and get her in the seat.

When I took her to the clinic for immunisations or to be weighed, other parents used to stare at us, which I found very distressing so our Health Visitor came to us instead.

Luckily the harness was 100% successful for Daisy who is now six and always dancing and loves her trampoline. Whilst it was distressing and upsetting at the time, we know how lucky we are that the pediatrician picked up the problem so early and that the first round of treatment worked.

Purdey

I started noticing it more often, analysing her left leg and wondering if it was shorter. Am I seeing things or it just the way she's stretching her cute little legs? I mentioned it to my husband and he said he'd noticed it too and to mention it in her eight-month check.

Then as I was carrying her on my hip, just like I always did, I heard a pop.

That night I was changing her nappy and something popped again, it was her left leg. Am I going mad? Did I just hear that? I called my husband and told him I was sure her hip popped. Purdey wasn't crying or in any pain in but I decided to go and see our GP.

The next day the doctor examined her left leg and said she could definitely feel something but told me usually it's just a case of wearing double nappies and we were referred to see a specialist. At that point I was oblivious to DDH, the severity of the condition and the treatment methods involved.

On the day of our appointment, the surgeon's nurse assessed Purdey, placing her legs in all different positions, listening out for the pop that I had been hearing since that day. I took her in for her X-ray and she was mesmerised by the big machine hovering over her little body.

We waited for what felt like a lifetime and were then called into an examination room where we were met by the registrar and two members of staff. There was an X-ray on the screen and the registrar wanted to check Purdey again, which made me think things must be OK. Then he invited us to sit down and said she had a dislocated left hip and she will need treatment.

That's when my whole world crumbled. My beautiful baby girl had DDH, her left hip was dislocated and she would need a procedure called a closed reduction to correct this. She would then be put into a cast for four months and then in a brace for another four months. The cast will start just below her nipples and go down both legs right down to her ankles....

I was in shock, my eyes were filling up, I was holding Purdey tighter than I've held her before "but she's my baby" I said through tears. How has this happened? I'm her mummy, I carried her for nine months, and did I do something? Was it my fault?

I was asked about my pregnancy and labour which were both healthy experiences. It had come to light a couple of weeks before that my brother-in-law had hip problems as a child, which we mentioned to the registrar.

Devastated was an understatement and I wanted to get out of that room as quick as possible. We left with a leaflet about DDH and the STEPS website and were told the date for Purdey's procedure would be within the next month.

That night we both read up on things but we were too exhausted to talk to each other. We were dealing with it in our own way. I felt so unbelievably alone. Even with all the family and friends we have, and as close we are as a couple, I felt alone and scared.

The month following was hard. Purdey started crawling which was bitter sweet as she was so proud and we would be taking that away from her when she went into a cast and as a mummy that was worst feeling in the world.

The one thing that really got to me was people sharing their experiences of knowing a friend's friend who had been through this and telling me "they were OK in the end". I know they were trying to help me but all it did was make me angry. I just wanted to shout at them "so it hasn't happened to you directly" and "you have no idea how I feel as a parent?"

I wanted to have patience but it was wearing thin. I was exhausted, I was hardly sleeping, and the op was going through my head. The vision of her being put to sleep was playing on my mind, would she wake up? What if something seriously went wrong when she was under anaesthetic? How was she going to react to this strange weight constantly attached her? I was stressed, my alopecia had retuned; I was feeling drained and alone.

My husband was so sweet, he did lots of research and I couldn't have coped without him. He's my rock and I needed him more than ever to keep reassuring me things were going to be ok.

Preparing for the operations was hard. What can she wear, who will we change her, will she fit in her car seat and the push-chair? Everything was going through my mind. But we got organised and did it all whilst getting ready to move house.

On the day of the operation, Purdey was first on the list and with no bottle allowed since the night before, we did all we could to keep her occupied. I was nervous but wasn't going to show it. I'd wait for her to be out of sight before I broke down.

After our surgeon drew a big black arrow on her left leg I took a picture of her and what a beautiful picture it was.

Purdey loved the ride down to theatre. Her cot was full of her teddies, a suitcase full of them to be precise, as I wanted to be sure she had her home comforts and smells around her.

I was dreading this moment. James and I had spoken about who was going to take her and hold her while she was put to sleep. As a mummy you feel very protective and want to be the one who makes everything OK. But in the same respect I didn't want James to feel like I was taking over but deep down I knew he didn't want to do it. I knew seeing his little girl in distress would break him.

We took dolly in with us and I held Purdey in my arms before she was placed in the hands of strangers. I prayed they would bring her back to me safely. James was waiting and gave me a huge hug and we went for a coffee and tried to kill time during the longest hour of our lives.

When we went up to recovery I couldn't walk fast enough. The next few hours were horrible as she was so unhappy and scared, but it got better. We stayed in hospital for two nights; she slept really well and coped amazingly.

We were discharged after having an MRI, which confirmed it had worked which was a massive relief. We put her in her new car seat but she cried most of the way home. It was going to be trial and error with the car seat but we found ways for her to be comfortable and safe. I was determined we were not going to become prisoners in our own home.

The next couple of days were spent practicing the nappy changes and getting her comfortable. We propped her up on a beanbag and would sit for hours passing her things to keep her occupied. I used a Hippy Chick seat, which was great as she was extremely heavy. It was hard physically and emotionally and the first ten days were horrible but it got better.

After eight weeks, she had her cast changed, which again was upsetting but this one was smaller and lighter, which was amazing as she felt closer to me and she loved it too. It also meant I could look to go back to work for a couple of days a week as my mum looked after her.

She moves more in this cast, she army crawls everywhere, rolls from front to back and back again and laughs when she does it. Her upper body strength is something else, her arms are big and when she is determined to reach for things she won't give up until she gets them.

With only five sleeps to go until the cast comes off, I admit I'm feeling scared and anxious. I'm worried about the results, has it worked? Will her legs look pitiful and weak? How's she going to adapt?

My biggest bit of advice is don't underestimate just how amazing your little one is and how amazing you are too. They cope and because you are a mummy you will do whatever it takes to make things right. I have days when I feel alone and tired and envious of parents with children who are walking but I remind myself Purdey has DDH, and nothing more. This will be sorted and one day she will be making up dances for me in the front room. And for that I am blessed.

Melissa

You were a hidden shock introduced to us having never met you before, you were unwanted, unnoticed and found hidden within our beautiful 'perfect' girl... then came the bigger shock of no quick fix, anaesthetics and a cast for 12 weeks?

What!

But we didn't even notice... she isn't different from her baby friends, the weight bearing might be just slower?

You held us in a time warp of what felt like never ending panic and waiting... you were used to hiding but when we had found/exposed you, you became a monster...this was the time where you nearly had us! But no, we wouldn't let that happen!

DDH you are the hidden thing which creeps up and changes everything, brings uncertainty, a future of worry and doubt, initiating us to the world of hospitals, casts, braces, equipment.

But DDH you have given us as much hope as you have taken, you have shown us how strong we are as a family, how brave we can be and how much we can rise to your challenge!

You have brought out the best in our girl, the smiles, the determination, the pure resilience, the acceptance, trust and easy going, loveable personality. She rocked her casts, she bravely accepted and got through these endless anaesthetics and cast changes, she didn't care if she smelt like a horse's stable due to leaking in her cast, she cheerfully waved to her brother in the bath when she couldn't join him, she flew high in a swing and sat on a horse all in the cast caused by you!

Oh and the day she came out, the 12 weeks were over, she waved her legs all the way home with the biggest smile ever. We are too aware of the fact that you're lurking round the corner, are you cooperating? Any bone growth? More surgery? But know this DDH we are ready for you! As a family we will meet whatever is to come and for that we can say THANK YOU to you as before we met you I had no idea we could take this on and how much strength my perfect little girl had to laugh her way through the majority of your visit!

Cameron

I was born in 1968 and diagnosed with bilateral DDH by a vigilant doctor whose daughter was wheelchair bound because of the condition. I was in traction and wooden splints for about eight weeks and then had yearly X-rays and check-ups until the age of seven.

When my sons were born, medical staff checked their hips and whilst my first son escaped, number two didn't. Cameron was born breech and was diagnosed with bilateral DDH. He was fitted with a Pavlik harness and adjusted straight away. Other than changing from cloth nappies to disposable ones we didn't have to adapt much. We were allowed to take the harness off for half an hour every second day for a bath and went to the hospital once a fortnight to have the harness checked and adjusted.

The harness stayed on for a three months and the final ultrasound showed good progress. The following year he had two check-ups and X-rays which showed his hips were developing well. He had a check-up at three and four years old. At that last appointment he was given the all clear, which was great, as we had already started the DDH journey with his baby brother.

Cameron is a sporty boy but tends to get knee and ankle injuries so he works with his physiotherapist to build up his core strength and hip muscles and we monitor his hip pain and gait. He is now 14 and wants a career in physio or sports science and is really interested in the musco/skeletal system.

I would say we coped with DDH well and were always given positive expectations to aim for.

Holly

On the day I was born in 1994, the midwife noted that my left hip was 'clicky' and whilst it was put on my birth report, no follow up appointment was made. At my six-week review my hips were examined but there was no mention of them being 'clicky'. A health visitor assessed me at nine months and my parents believe that my hips weren't even checked.

At about a year and seven months old, when I started walking, my parents noticed I was limp. I went to see a GP who said I had a twisted pelvis and I was referred to a surgeon. The surgeon examined me and said I limped because of a shorter left leg and an X-ray showed I had DDH/CDH in my left hip but my right hip was normal.

I was admitted to hospital for an open reduction of my left hip and then placed in a cast. Five weeks later I had a Derotational Varus Osteotomy where they broke my femur and put it back in a different position, held in place with bolts and plates. As the hospital had not conducted this type of surgery on someone so young before, adult size plates were used but because they were too big they stuck out of my skin. I was still put in plaster again.

Three months after I was taken out of plaster and my X-rays were shown to be satisfactory. 10 months later the plates were removed.

When I was about five my doctor put in his notes that I needed a pelvis osteotomy, yet nothing was done. His solution was watch and wait. We did this until I was 10 at which point I was referred to a new surgeon at a hospital which specialises in orthopaedics. I had an arthogram and it was then decided to finally have my pelvis/shelf osteotomy; only five years late.

I remember this operation and recovery so well as I was placed in a huge plaster from my chest to my toes. I left hospital after a week and went home via ambulance because I was too big to fit in our car. I couldn't fit through a doorway without being turned on my side and both my parents had to take six weeks off work to look after me.

I couldn't get up the stairs so I had a bed in the living room. I had to be turned from my front to my back regularly to circulate the air, and going to the toilet was a complete nightmare as we couldn't get access to the correct equipment.

I missed a lot of school and as I only managed to get a private tutor for one session my mum taught me. She was great and my education hasn't suffered at all. I had a wheelchair bed, which apparently looked horrendous, but it meant I wasn't trapped in the house for six weeks.

Looking back I'm not sure how I coped as it was incredibly tough but my parents tried their best to keep me entertained and positive. My plaster was removed six weeks later. I had two weeks intensive physiotherapy and by the end of this period I was walking again with the aid of frame.

To be honest, support after that was pretty poor. I struggled with walking long distances (and still do) but it was a real fight to get physiotherapy and I got sick and tired of being told I needed to be more active. I was trying my hardest, but as I person who has never enjoyed physical activity I struggled. I tried wearing a wedge in my shoe to make up the leg length difference, but I gave up with that as I felt it was making no difference. In some ways I regret that operation. I know I had no choice but it honestly seems like nothing has been right since.

At 18, I left home and went to Liverpool to study Geography and I'm now 21, in my final year and living with my boyfriend. Health wise, I'm not great and in the past year I've been diagnosed with Trochanteric Bursistis in my left hip, which I have steroid injections for, as well as osteoarthritis.

I've lost an incredible amount of confidence due to the deterioration of my hip and suffered from depression. There were times when I couldn't physically leave my flat for the pain. I stopped wanting to dress or put effort into my appearance and just couldn't see a light at the end of the tunnel. I'm getting through it but it's a challenge.

Daisy P

Daisy was born in February 2009, our first baby, a beautiful healthy girl. She was found to have a 'clicky hip', at her post-birth check-up the following day. I'd heard about them, my brother had had one but we didn't think much of it, she was perfect. We were told to wait for a scan date and we took our little bundle home.

We had no idea how long we were supposed to wait, and with a now more hectic life and newborn we forgot all about it.

She finally had an X-ray at five months old and we were told the devastating news that Daisy had bilateral DDH. Both of her hips were dislocated, she had very shallow sockets and she was immediately put into a Pavlik Harness. It was a massive shock for us, we went home and cried, and cuddled and immediately searched the Internet for more information, help and this is how we found the STEPS website.

When the shock subsided, we realised we weren't alone, that many children have DDH and we even met up with a local family whose daughter's hips had been fixed using the harness.

We started to feel a lot stronger and more positive, and despite the horrible looking harness, which was pretty grim after just two weeks, life went on and we even took her to two festivals in it!

Sadly, the harness didn't work for us, and after two failed closed reductions in the following months, she had an open reduction at 10 months old. She wore a dreaded spica cast for 12 weeks but we all coped brilliantly, especially Daisy who was soon rolling over and crawling around in it. Stuffing nappies inside it, sleek taping it and trying to get hold of essential non-absorbent cotton wool (like gold dust in the local NHS Trust) was hard work at times. She smelt like the bottom of a rabbit hutch for the last two weeks, but time flew by. She even started nursery in the spica and had her first birthday in it.

Daisy's right hip is now fixed and stable but she's had another open reduction and a pelvic osteotomy to build up her socket on the left side. She's been in two more spicas and a metal brace but whatever DDH throws at her, she keeps smiling. She needs more work to help fix her left hip, but I know she will take it all in her stride. For us, and her little sister, it might be slightly harder.

Chapter 13: Equipment and resources

When you have a child with DDH, your home will probably need some additions and changes to accommodate a cast and ensure they are as comfortable and happy as possible.

My advice would not be to go out and buy everything straight away but to wait until your child has had their treatment so you can see the angle and position of their harness or cast. I hope these ideas will help make life easier for your child, you and your family.

Beanbags, pillows and wedges

For many, a beanbag, or two, is a spica lifesaver. Today there is a wide range of products on the market with many retailers selling various options and these include Amazon, Argos, Dunelm Mill, www.greatbeanbags.com, John Lewis and www.fatboy.com.

The Doomoo, Bambeano and Poddle Pod are some of the most popular ones.

Doomoo

The Doomoo seat is an adaptable, multi-functional beanbag that is suitable from birth up to 30kg. The combination of micro balls and an extra soft stretch material, mean these flexible beanbags are soft and malleable making them perfect for harnesses and casts. They come in a range of colours in either a dream cotton or fleece finish and are machine washable at 30°C. They have an adjustable three-point harness and there is also an additional arch you can buy, which is great for keeping babies alert and occupied. Doomoo also sells multi-functional cushions that could be helpful for comfortable breast-feeding and sitting positions. Prices start at around £100 and details can be seen at www.doomoo.be

Bambeano beanbag

Similar in function to the Doomoo, the Bambeano beanbag has a lower price point at around £45. This model molds to the shape of your child's body and allows them to be fully supported in a semi-upright position so they can see the world around them. It is light, so easy to take from room to room, as well as convenient for popping in the car if you are visiting people. Details can be seen at www.bambeano.co.uk

Poddle Pod

Some parents I spoke to found the Poddle Pod very helpful. This weight activated snuggle nest is made of hypo allergenic, anti-fungal hollow-fibre filling and covered in 100% cotton. The Pod is not only comfortable, but breathable too and is a perfect resting place for a child in a spica. Details can be seen at www.poddlepod.com

V-Pillows

There are a wide range of v-pillows available on the market from many retailers and at various price points. The main aim of these is provide additional support and make your child comfortable. Argos, Amazon, John Lewis, Marks & Spencer and many other retailers sell these at reasonable prices.

Wedges

Depending on the setting of your cast and comfort of your child, you can use wedges to help them settle. Many come at an 11° angle to retain the body's natural posture and shape. They can help relieve pain and aches and offer comfort and relief. Amazon and www.betterlifehealthcare.com are good places to find these.

Pushchairs and prams
If you find you are in the position of needing a new pushchair, one of the best ideas is to go to a large John Lewis or Mothercare and try out models on display. It is a case of finding a model that works for your child and their cast. Popular options include:

- Baby Jogger City Mini
- Babyzen YoYo Stroller
- Bugaboo Frog
- Emmaljunga Twin Nitro double buggy
- Graco Ugo
- Jane Pro
- Mamas and Papas Armadillo
- Mamas and Papas Luna
- Mamas and Papas Sola
- Mamas and Papas Urbo
- Maclaren Major Elite Pushchair
- Maclaren Techno XT
- Micralite Fastfold Superlite Stroller
- Mothercare Nanu Stroller
- Silver Cross Pop
- Phil & Teds (my personal success story)
- Quinny Xtra

You can buy these at most major retailers and online. As costs do mount up, it might be worth seeing if family, friends or second hand sites (eBay and Gumtree) have one for sale.

Wheelchairs
For older and bigger children, a wheelchair will probably be required.

The 'Chunc' offers a post-operative mobility solution for children and young people in hip spica casts. The leg supports and backrest can fit the most awkward position created by those clever doctors and it allows continued participation in social, educational, home and therapy environments.

This is not a cheap option but a sanity saver for many and can be rented for the duration of the cast time plus it looks pretty cool so don't worry too much about stares! Full details can be seen at www.chunc.com

Car seats

Car seats can be a battle but where there's a will, there's a 'safe' way. For many, their original car seats simply aren't up to the job of holding a child in a spica. The main thing with getting this essential bit of kit right is finding a seat that is wide enough and deep enough; easy right?

The In-Car Safety Centre has, for more than 25 years, provided suitable seating to meet the 'special needs' of all children and they are 'the experts' when it comes to spica casts where the options are limited.

2-Way Elite CDH Modified (Britax)

This car seat has been specifically adapted for children in a spica. It can only be used rearward facing when in its adapted form as this significantly reduces the load weight on both the child and the harness in the event of an accident.

The seat is supplied ready for use, fully adapted, and a manual is sent with the seat and 'how to fit' videos may be viewed on the website. Specification details:

- Installation with two or three point seatbelt
- Five point safety harness with three setting height adjustable harness
- ONLY to be used rear facing when the child is in the cast/brace and rear facing tether straps are supplied
- Recline function
- For children under 18 months, the additional head support is recommended

The 2-Way Elite will accommodate most children in a spica and there is an extended crotch strap and additional padding to lift the bottom and support the back. In-Car Safety offers this seat

in two ways, through a loan scheme or through outright purchase.

For children who do not fit into this seat, there is also the
option of using the E-Z On Harness. For more details about
both of these options and the loan offer, speak to Simon Bel-
lamy, In-Car Safety on 02890 742052 or go to www.incarsafe-
tycentre.co.uk.

Maxi-Cosi Opal HD

Another option comes from Maxi-Cosi (part of the Dorel
group) which has adapted its Opal car seat for children in a hip
spica cast and developed the Maxi-Cosi Opal HD.

This chair offers extra space for the legs and support for the
back, even when the cast has been set wide. It is installed in the
car using the seat belt and can be used rear facing up to 13kg,
before being turned forward facing.

The seat offers normality with its comfy, padded seats, an
extra support pillow for younger babies and recline adjustments.
This is an easy to use seat that has a compact design, which fits
all cars as well as having a side protection system for optimal
protection in side impact collisions.

There is a great loan scheme for this with STEPS and details
can be seen at www.maxi-cosi.co.uk and www.steps-char-
ity.org.uk/How-We-Help/hip-spica-car-seats.html

Highchairs

When your child is in their cast you may find that they need to
use a different highchair so they fit and are safe. Whilst this can
be frustrating, and expensive, it is worth the investment because
as well as being able to eat here they can also colour, craft, play
games and watch TV. Here are some popular choices:

Chicco Happy Snack Highchair

Many parents like and use this highchair due to the fact it is
lightweight, the large tray has four positions and the seat features

a rigid crotch strap and five-point safety harness. The seat cushion is removable for cleaning.

This can be purchased from retailers such as Argos, Amazon and Mothercare.

Chicco Polly Highchair

This is also a very popular choice. It has a large double padded seat that offers great support and comfort and has two layers so those with older children, or a large spica, have extra space without compromising comfort. It has an adjustable, removable tray which means it can be used for direct table use. There are open sides so good for wide casts and we used this with Lucas in his frog cast but did have to make a slit in the side of the fabric.

This can be purchased from retailers such as Argos, Amazon and Mothercare.

Nuna Zaaz

The Nuna Zaaz highchair has designer looks and a clever, modular system that means the size and design are totally customisable. The tray, armbar and footrest can be removed making it potentially suitable for use with a spica as it offers a number of configurations. The air-foam cushion offers a comfortable seat and there is a five-point harness, featuring a quick-click release button, which can be changed to a three-point harness as your child grows.

This can be purchased in the UK at John Lewis and details can be seen at www.nuna.eu

Stokke Tripp Trapp

The original Tripp Trapp revolutionised the world of highchairs and with added cushions and padding, its lack of sides make it another option for children in spicas (www.stokke.com)

Travel highchairs

Travel highchairs can be a cost-effective solution for aiding life in a spica cast. Depending on how your child's cast has been set it can make meal and play times easier, it is perfect for using on the go and when travelling and the harnesses offered by many ensure your child is safe and comfortable. Some products worth looking at include:

Bumbo

These handy, sturdy, low level seats aren't advisable in their purchased state, but many parents find that cutting larger holes from the original legs make a perfect seat for spica kids. Some of the new models come with trays too making it a great activity and eating station at an affordable price. www.bumbo.com

JoJo Super Lightweight Pocket Highchair

This is a very handy piece of kit that allows your child to sit at the table to eat and play safely. Although I wouldn't leave them unsupervised whilst in it. It isn't expensive and with the help of a pillow or two it is a reported lifesaver for many. www.jojomamanbebe.co.uk

The Munchkin

The Munchkin travel child booster seat is a convenient booster seat that can be easily secured to a chair; it is simple to clean and features a harness for safety. Available from Argos, Amazon, ASDA, Tesco and other leading retailers.

Polar Gear Baby Booster Seat

This great seat is lightweight and simple to attach to any standard chair. It has a five-point safety harness and adjustable straps so you can get the position just right for your child. It has a wipe clean, removable cushioned seat and folds down and clips shut for convenient transportation so great if you are going out. Available from Amazon, JoJo Maman Bebe, Mothercare and other outlets.

The Tot Seat

The Tot Seat is loved by many parents with kids in a cast. It is made of soft fabric and adapts to fit chairs of varying heights, includes al fresco fasteners for rounded, metal-framed chairs, and has a secure wide strap to create a back support on open-backed chairs. www.totseat.com

Clothes

Dressing a child in a Pavlik harness or spica cast can be a challenge, but with a little knowledge and creativity, it can be done. Going for bigger dresses, colourful leggings and adapted vests, you can have a cool looking, comfortable child whatever situation you are in.

Buying items in charity shops and on eBay and Gumtree in bigger sizes means you can cut and adapt them and it doesn't matter. Chapter 3 has extensive details about clothing if your child is in a Pavlik harness and if they are in a spica cast, Chapter 7 is full of handy advice.

DDH specific clothing sites:
- Hip-Pose (UK) www.hip-pose.co.uk
- Kiek Hip Wear (The Netherlands) www.kiekhipwear.co.uk

Other sites I love include:
- Amazon and Etsy have some great bargains and offers.
- Babykind - www.babykind.co.uk/mylittlelegs-legwarmers.htm
- Tiny Nippers - www.tinynippers.co.uk/clothing/leg-warmers

Slings

Parents can use baby slings to carry their children whilst in a spica cast. Obviously the cast adds weight and bulk, so it is very important that not only is your child safe but also you are comfortable and are not going to injury your back, muscles or shoulders. Remember; a healthy parent, both physically and mentally, is a happy, helpful parent. If your baby has a cast with a bar between the legs, it is unlikely this will be relevant for you. Slings that have been recommended by parents include:

Boba

The Boba Wrap is a versatile stretchy wrap that snuggles your baby close and offers a variety of carrying positions. The wrap is easy to use and free of buckles and straps, you will be wrapping in confidence within minutes so your baby is comfortable in their spica and you are too. www.boba.com

Ergobaby

This sling has a padded waist belt that ensures baby's weight is evenly distributed between your hips and shoulders while the adjustable, padded shoulder straps provide you with ultimate comfort. www.ergobaby.co.uk

Hippy Chick

Not a sling but I felt this was the best place for this handy piece of kit. Specifically designed to address adult back pain, the Hippychick Hipseat has a firm shelf for the child to sit on and supports their weight from underneath. The back remains straight and the child is tucked into the chest on whichever side is more comfortable for the wearer, making it perfectly safe solution for carrying a child in a spica – their weight permitting. www.hippy-chick.com

Manduca

These are soft structured carriers with an ergonomic waist belt and padded shoulder straps that redistribute the weight from the shoulders to the hips. The integrated head support can be folded away in a pocket and they can be used for front, hip and back carries so you can see what works best with your child. www.manduca-baby-carrier.eu

Moby Wraps

The design of the MobyTM Wrap uses your entire back, as well as your shoulders, to carry the weight of your baby. It has no buckles or fasteners; it is simply a wide piece of fabric that is wrapped over both shoulders. It is easy to adjust and the convenient one size (5.5 meters) fits nearly all adults and many parents find it does work with a spica. www.mobywrap.com

Tutal

This sling has dual-adjustment straps to allow for the perfect fit, additional leg openings and shoulder padding as well as a large pocket on the contouring hip belt. www.tulababycarriers.com

Many of these models can be bought direct from the manufacturer, but also at Amazon, www.lovetobenatural.co.uk and www.itsaslingthing.co.uk, which also rents out slings.

You can also search for local sling libraries and they rent out models, which can really help save money and prevent you buying the wrong thing. Details can be seen at ukslinglibraries.wordpress.com and www.babywearing.co.uk

It is advisable to check use of baby carriers and slings with your doctor before using them just to be sure.

Spica tables

There are many takes on the spica table, both home and professionally made, but the essence of them all is to offer a child a safe place to 'sit' and eat, play, watch TV and give them a little independence and feeling of normality.

Smirthwaite has designed a range of products aimed at children in spica casts (www.smirthwaite.co.uk):

STEPS Hip Spica chair was designed in collaboration with STEPS and this adjustable, supportive chair provides safe seating for children from eight months who are in a hip spica cast. The chair comes complete with pelvic strap, shoulder harness and tray.

The Multi-Adjustable Hip Spica chair is available in three sizes and is ideal for children from the age of 18 months up to young adult using spica casts. The front section of the chair has a storage area and the back fully reclines for a more comfortable position.

The Portable Hip Spica chair is a lightweight, spacing saving model that can easily be taken apart and is perfect for transporting in a car. Suitable for children aged 12 months to three years old, it is supplied with a five-point harness and quick release tray as standard.

Smirthwaite offers the Portable Hip Spica table on a rental service at a cost of £40.00 per month for a minimum of three months. The first payment is taken by card and then a standing order is set up. www.smirthwaite.co.uk

Hip Rocker

The standard hip-Rocker Chair is suitable from six months to three years. This rocking chair and table has been specially designed for a child in a hip spica cast by parents who looked at the issues they faced with their own daughter.

The chair is 60cm in width 90cm in length and up to 60cm in height. It has anti-bacterial easy wipe clean table top and up standing edges so that toys do not fall off. This product allows a child to carry on having some level of independence, can even be personalised and comes in a variety of colours and sizes making it less medical and more fun. www.hip-rocker.org

As well as being purchased direct from the manufacturers, spica tables can sometimes be loaned from your hospital or you can try STEPS and social media forums to buy or loan them from other families.

If you, or someone you know, is great at DIY, it is possible to adapt furniture to create your own spica table. A quick 'DIY spica tables' search on Google brings up some great ideas. Be sure it is made well, it is safe and sturdy and suitable for use.

The International Hip Dysplasia Institute has instructions for making a table: www.hipdysplasia.org/wp-content/up-loads/2011/01/Gavins-Spica.pdf

Medical kit

I would advise finding a local chemist where you can get to know the pharmacy team and know that you can get the items your child needs quickly and easily and ask for help if you need it. If you find this isn't possible good websites include:

- Amazon
- Boots.com
- healthandcare.co.uk
- farmaline.co.uk

Basic equipment for your medical kit include:

- Antiseptic hand gel and wipes
- Cotton wool
- Emollient creams and Sudocrem
- General first aid kit to cover all eventualities
- Medical gloves
- Medicine spoons / syringes for medicines
- Plaster assortment
- Nail or toothbrush for cleaning the cast
- Clean, sharp scissors
- Thermometer

I would also buy a torch and keep it handy so you can check the skin inside the cast.

Medicines

- Calpol (paracetamol) for pain relief as needed
- Nurofen (Ibuprofen) for pain relief as needed but check with your surgeon or GP with regard to ongoing use with this
- Rescue Remedy gummy stars and Recuse Remedy for you!

- Movicol for constipation; take direction from your doctor on this

Tapes and padding

There are a wide range of tapes and padding on the market that are compatible for use with spica casts. Chemists and online retailers are the best places to get these but some hospitals do provide a limited supply when you are discharged.

Cellona is an adhesive padding that is great to use on hard cast edges.

Cohesive sports bandage sticks to itself and not to skin or hair and we found it helpful. It is easy to use and because it adheres to itself you do not need pins or tape and it looks good and hides marks and dirt without trapping the smell.

Gamgee Gauze Tissue is a thick layer of highly absorbent cotton wool enclosed in an absorbent cotton gauze cover. It's great for under-cast padding and particularly useful for preventing pressure sores.

Moleskin is a handy stick-on padding that protects against painful friction and cushions the skin from the cast. There are many brands out there so it is a case of working out what is best for your child and their cast.

Sleek Tape is waterproof adhesive strapping and great for using around the edges of the spica. It is strong and pretty reliable but also had a slight stretch that allows it to mold to the cast just make sure there are no sharp edges to irritate skin.

Nappies and toileting

- Disposable or cloth nappies in various sizes and strengths
- Incontinence pads
- Sanitary towels

Funnels allow older girls to keep their independence and saves blushes whilst in casts:

- Whiz Freedom - whizproducts.co.uk
- Lady Funnel - www.beambridgemedical.com

- Shewee - www.shewee.com

There are also a variety of bedpans and urinals on the market that are ideal for bedside use or when out and about or at school. They are hygienic and designed for use whilst sitting, standing or lying down. The female adaptor is easy to fit and the snap on lid helps prevent accidental spillages on casts.

www.welcomemobility.co.uk is a good place to find a wide range of these products.

When using them to start with just ensure there are no spills on the cast, a couple of practice runs might be needed.

Washing and cleaning
Cast Cooler
Some parents do use a CastCooler whilst their child is in a spica. This device provides relief from an itchy, hot, sweaty cast as it quickly cools, dries and freshens the cast. CastCoolers can be purchased from www.cover-my-cast.com

Bath time
These are some basic essentials that will make life easier:
- A stock of clean flannels or sponges
- A stock of clean towels and extra towels if you are washing hair over the kitchen sink with your child on the units
- A mild, organic soap or body wash
- A mild, tear free shampoo
- A tangle tamer hairbrush and spray in lotion (hair gets very matted when a child spends a lot of time lying on their backs)
- An inflatable shampoo ring or tray for easier hair washing; good place to buy these is www.welcomemobility.co.uk
- Moisturisers
- A pot of bubbles for distraction purposes
- A second pair of hands and a great deal of patience

Cast cleaning materials

As already mentioned, you cannot wash casts. By the pure nature of the beast, and kids being kids, they will get dirty and probably smelly.

Below are some deodorising ideas and your doctor, or local chemist, can help too, another reason to have that relationship with them.

- Baking soda - a little baking soda can help to dry up some moisture and cover some of the smell of a stinky cast. Gently powder the cast with a small amount of baking soda
- EcoClinic is an environmentally friendly odour neutraliser based on natural enzymes
- Febreze
- Limone ostomy deodorant spray
- Lavender, eucalyptus and tea tree oils can be used very sparingly and not close to skin
- Neutradol

Scar care

As already mentioned, there is a chance your child will have a scar(s) as a result of their surgery. These can be sensitive but do fade in time and they are a part of the healing process.

Good products to massage into the skin, once your child is ready and there is no broken skin, include:

- Bio-Oil for scars, stretch marks and dehydrated skin
- Trilogy Certified Organic Rosehip Oil
- Palmer's Cocoa Butter Formula Skin Therapy Oil

Mobility and equipment websites

There are many websites that sell a range of specialist products you might like to try. From bedpans and wedges to funnels and hair washing pods, below are some of the sites that might help you:

www.betterlifehealthcare.com
Betterlife is a part of the Lloyds Pharmacy group and sells a wide range of products to help with everyday tasks like bathing, dressing and generally helping to support everyday life.

www.jenx.com
Jenx sells therapeutic products for children with special needs.

www.livingmadeeasy.org.uk
Living Made Easy has a whole section on equipment designed to assist your child with daily living activities as well as play and learning.

www.localmobility.co.uk
Local Mobility sells a comprehensive range of products to help with everyday living.

www.welcomemobility.co.uk
Welcome Mobility has a great children's section, especially useful for older kids looking to maintain an element of independence. They have a variety of easy to use, hygienic bed pans and portable urinals for boys and girls.

www.torc2.com
torc2 Ltd is a UK based company developing a range of medical splinting devices that offer many advantages over current systems.

Financial support
Many people find that taking care of a child with DDH and the multiple appointments, hospital visits and stays mean an increase in expenses and also the potential loss of earnings.

During your child's DDH journey you, and your child, may be entitled to some financial assistance and concessions to help with the increase in living and travelling costs that are normally associated with caring for a child with disabilities.

There is help out there for you so do not despair if you are finding the cost of car parking, petrol, hospital canteen meals and hotel stays adding up. There is no shame in admitting you need financial support. If you don't it will simply eat away at you and add to the pressure you might already be experiencing.

Some of these benefits are means tested, whilst others are based on the needs of your child and it does seem that this varies a lot from case to case and in different areas of the country.

The process can seem very daunting, particularly when it comes to completing the forms, and it could take time for claims to be processed but if it helps, it is worth the time and effort and will hopefully ease some of the additional pressures you face.

Government funding

Disability Living Allowance for Children (DLA) is a tax-free benefit for children under 16 to help with the extra costs caused by long-term ill health or a disability.

Carer's Allowance is extra money to help you look after someone with substantial caring needs. You may also be able to claim Carer's Credit, which means there won't be any gaps in your National Insurance record if you have to take on caring responsibilities. Other benefits include:

- Working and Child Tax Credit
- Vehicle Road Tax Exemption
- Vehicle Purchase (Motability)
- Blue House Adaptations (Disabled Facilities Grant)
- VAT relief on products and services

Blue Badge parking scheme

The Blue Badge parking scheme offers a range of parking concessions for people with severe mobility problems who find using public transport difficult. When you have a child in a heavy cast being able to park close to the places you need to visit is really helpful. Blue Badge guidelines are as follows:

Children aged 0 – three years
Children under three who need bulky medical equipment that cannot be carried around (e.g. a spica cast) might be entitled to a Blue Badge but this will expire on their third birthday.

Whilst the badge can help work with parking restrictions and limit the amount of walking needed to access services, it is for your child not the car. If you do get a badge, ensure your child is in the car when it is displayed.

Children aged over three
The general guide to the Blue Badge being awarded to children over the age of three, is that they need to have been awarded a mobility component at the higher rate of DLA, which is awarded over the age of three and for permanent conditions.

The Blue Badge scheme is run by local councils and they can let you know details for your area.

For more information about all of these and more go to www.gov.uk or call The Disability Living Allowance helpline 0345 712 3456.

Hospital help and funding
One of the best places to start is at your hospital and not only should your medical team have information but the Patient Advice and Liaison Service (PALS) should be of help too. Help can include free or reduced hospital parking and free meals for parents.

DDH specific charities
SPICA WARRIOR - www.spicawarrior.org
STEPS - www.steps-charity.org.uk
IHD - hipdysplasia.org

Other helpful charities
www.avncharity.org.uk

Avascular Necrosis AVN Charity UK is spreading awareness, understanding, support and research into this rare bone condition.

www.cashforkids.uk.com
Cash for Kids lends a helping hand to disabled and disadvantaged children aged 0 to 18 years by means of grants awarded to go towards buying specialist equipment in order to enhance their quality of life.

www.caudwellchildren.com
Caudwell Children provides family support services, equipment, treatment and therapies for disabled children and their families across the UK.

www.adviceguide.org.uk
Citizen's Advice Bureau

www.cafamily.org.uk
Contact a Family provides information, advice and support and brings together families so they can support each other.

www.child-disability.co.uk
Child Disability Help offers a wide range of information and support.

www.disability-grants.org
Disability grants information.

www.disabilityrightsuk.org
Disability rights information.

www.dlf.org.uk
DLF is a national charity providing impartial advice, information and training on independent living since 1969.

www.familyfund.org.uk
Family Fund is the UK's largest provider of grants to low-income families raising disabled and seriously ill children and young people. They can help with essential items such as clothing but also consider grants for sensory toys, computers and family breaks.

www.familyandchildcaretrust.org
The Family and Childcare Trust works with the National Association of Family Information Services and represents a network of local Family Information Services to support families across England, Wales and Scotland.

www.motability.co.uk
Motablity is a national charity which aims to help disabled people with their personal mobility.

www.marthacare.org.uk
Martha Care is a charity set up by parents for parents and families when they find themselves in hospital with a very ill or injured child for a few days or longer.

www.moneyadviceservice.org.uk
Money Advice Service

www.portage.org.uk
Portage is a home-visiting educational service for pre-school children with additional support needs and their families.

www.rmhc.org.uk
Ronald McDonald House Charities provides free 'home away from home' accommodation for families with children in 14 specialist children's hospitals across the UK. Parents can be with their children in minutes but have some of the emotional and financial stresses associated with hospital life taken away from them for a while.

www.scope.org.uk
Scope, a disability charity, has a huge amount of easy to understand information about benefits and issues relating to disability.

www.sibs.org.uk
Sibs is the only UK charity representing the needs of siblings of disabled people. Siblings have a lifelong need for information; they often experience social and emotional isolation, and have to cope with difficult situations.

www.wellchild.org.uk
WellChild is a national charity offering excellent care and support for children and families with long-term and complex health conditions.

www.newlifecharity.co.uk
The Newlife Foundation offers a range of help, information and support for the family and carers of disabled and ill children.

www.samaritans.org
The Samaritans are available 24 hours a day to provide confidential emotional support for people who are experiencing feelings of distress, despair or suicidal thoughts.

Medical organisations
www.bscos.org.uk
British Society for Children's Orthopaedic Surgery

www.boa.ac.uk
British Orthopaedic Association

www.nhs.uk/carersdirect/
To speak to someone at Carers Direct call 0300 123 1053 from 9am to 8pm Monday to Friday, and 11am to 4pm at weekends.

www.nhs.uk
National Health Service (UK)

Experts in this book
Dr. Amanda Gummer
Research Psychologist Specialising in Child Development
www.fundamentallychildren.com

Dr. Rachel Andrew
Clinical Psychologist
www.drrachelandrew.com

Professor N M P Clarke ChM, DM, FRCS.
Consultant Orthopaedic Surgeon
www.southampton.ac.uk/medicine/about/staff/nmpc.page

Eve Menezes Cunningham
Holistic Therapist and Founder of the Feel Better Every Day
Consultancy
www.feelbettereveryday.co.uk

Fi Star-Stone
Child Care Expert and Broadcaster
www.childcareisfun.co.uk

Mr. Hashemi-Nejad
Consultant Orthopaedic Surgeon at Royal National Orthopaedic Hospital
www.rnoh.nhs.uk/health-professionals/consultants/mr-aresh-
hashemi-nejad

Jenny Tschiesche BSc Hons, Dip(ION) FdSc BANT)
Leading nutrition expert
www.lunchboxdoctor.com

Books

The Parents' Guide to Hip Dysplasia by Betsy Miller

A Guide for Adults with Hip Dysplasia by Dr. Sophie West & Denise Sutherland

Hope Hip Hippo by Gina Jay

Going to the Hospital by Anna Civardi

Maisy Goes to Hospital by Lucy Cousins

Topsy and Tim: Go to Hospital by Jean Adamso

Peppa Pig: Peppa Goes to Hospital: My First Storybook by Ladybird

Blogging for happiness: a guide to improving positive mental health (and wealth) from your blog by Ellen Arnison

Blogs

abbysbilateralhipdysplasiastory.blogspot.co.uk
dramaticallyhip.com
emmaand3.com
happyhips.webs.com
hipbuddies.com
hip-baby.org
hiphiphoorayhips.blogspot.com.au
hiphipboo.wordpress.com
hopethehiphippo.com
justbecauseilove.co.uk
livingwithhipdysplasia.wordpress.com
mummaplusthree.com
themummycode.wordpress.com
northernmum.com
onehipworld.blogspot.co.uk
walkingwithlily.weebly.com

Facebook pages and support
Children Facing Surgery or Spica Casts
www.facebook.com/groups/Hiptoddlers/

DDH Support Worldwide
www.facebook.com/groups/ddhsupportworldwide

Healthy Hips Australia
www.facebook.com/healthyhipsaustralia

Hip Dysplasia Awareness Group
www.facebook.com/groups/11256957586

Hip Dysplasia Baby
www.facebook.com/HipDysplasiaBaby

Hip Dysplasia Awareness Ireland
www.facebook.com/pages/Developmental-Hip-Dysplasia-awareness-Ireland

Hip Dysplasia Awareness/Hips Don't Lie
www.facebook.com/hipchica

Hip Dysplasia In Babies (clicky hips or CHD, DDH)
www.facebook.com/groups/HipDysplasiaInBabies

Hip Dysplasia, Total Hip Replacements & Hip & Knee Problems
www.facebook.com/groups/111645505661430

Hip Hip Hooray DDH – Australia
www.facebook.com/hiphiphoorayddh
www.hiphiphoorayddh.org
Twitter - @hiphiphoorayddh

Hip Kid Story
www.facebook.com/hipkidstory
www.hipkidstory.com

Parents who have kids with DDH
www.facebook.com/groups/1547639968836619

Spica Warrior
www.facebook.com/pages/Spica-Warrior/1638707209742941

There's Nothing Hip About Hip Dysplasia
www.facebook.com/TheresNothingHipAboutDysplasia

Index

214

NELL JAMES PUBLISHERS

www.nelljames.co.uk

250+ fundraising ideas for your charity, society, school and PTA by Paige Robinson

**Blogging for happiness
A guide to improving positive mental health (and wealth) from your blog** by Ellen Arnison

Birth trauma: A guide for you, your friends and family to coping with post-traumatic stress disorder following birth by Kim Thomas

How to overcome fear of driving: The road to driving confidence by Joanne Mallon

Survival guide for new parents: Pregnancy, birth and the first year by Charlie Wilson

Test tubes and testosterone: A man's journey into infertility and IVF by Michael Saunders

**Toddlers: an instruction manual
A guide to surviving the years one to four**
by Joanne Mallon

The Volunteer Fundraiser's Handbook
by Jimmy James